Chakra Healing For Beginners:

A Complete Guide To Balance The Power Of Chakra Through Self-Healing Techniques In Order To Attract Positive Energy And Discover The Benefits Of Your Third Eye Awakening.

Table of Contents:

Introduction

Congratulations on purchasing *"Chakra Healing For Beginners: A Complete Guide To Balance The Power Of Chakra Through Self-Healing Techniques In Order To Attract Positive Energy And Discover The Benefits Of Your Third Eye Awakening."* and thank you for doing so.

Now, we would like to start with this message: chakra meditation, or even the existence of chakra, should grace the top of the list when you're trying to achieve holistic health. In this book, we will talk all there is to know about how our mind and body may be two different categories, but the act of balancing your chakra system can bring about amazing benefits for both aspects. You see, most of the time, when you are trying to better yourself, you are only either improving your physical health or your mental health, but never the two. If you feel like there is an improvement as to both your physical and mental health, chances are that it's very minimal. So, what are you supposed to do? Well, the chakra framework may come in handy. We explained here as to what the chakra system is, what are chakras, their purpose in our life, how balancing each of the energy centers in our body can bring about goodness and salvation in our life, and so much more including techniques, meditation poses, tools and instruments to further help you achieve a well-balanced chakra system, and color and gemstone correspondences that are often associated with each chakra point.

If you have been attempting to live a good life but mental anxiety or physical impairments have been in your way lately, you may want to change how you approach the situation. In this book, we will show you how to properly assess your chakra system and how you can open each one of them up. Moreover, we'll also clarify some of the misconceptions about chakra meditative practice. The truth is that meditation has been around for hundreds and thousands of years, yet the real reason why it is still being practiced today is that it works!

Whether you are already an advanced student or simply starting out on your chakra meditative journey, this book would be your perfect companion on the road to achieving holistic health. Without further ado, proceed to the next chapters of this book and start your learning session.

Chapter 1:
Getting Started: Learning All About Chakras

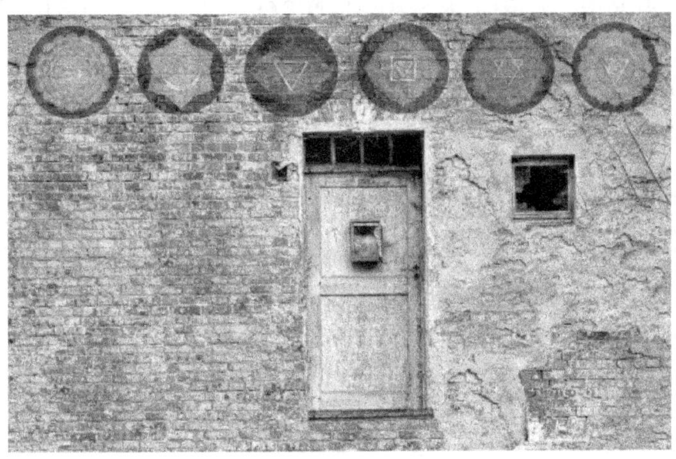

You may have already heard of the word "chakra" from various sources, but it doesn't mean that you are able to comprehend its definition. There has been a lot of debate regarding this topic, most of which focuses on whether there are actually chakra points and if these are the keys to attaining a healthy mind and body. Well, even though we can safely assume that you're reading this book because you believe in its power, it is still proper to talk more about how it came to be.

Let's start with the terminologies; the word "chakra" in Sanskrit connotes a wheel. It is often utilized in different auxiliary, subordinate, and symbolical faculties. The image of the wheel is also used in many other beliefs. In Buddhism, it portrays the wheel of life and death. Moreover, it depicts the very first lesson in time where Buddha talked about how one of his tenets was the Dhammachakkappavattana Sutta. Moreover, it was Chakka that was considered as the Pali version for the Sanskrit Chakra, which Professor Rhys Davids gracefully renders as "to set rolling the regal chariot wheel of an all-inclusive domain of truth and honesty." Do keep in mind that this is the true meaning which the articulation passes on to any Buddhist enthusiast; however, the strict interpretation of these words is "the turning of the wheel of the law." The wheel of the law pertains to the Dharmachakra. The exceptional utilization of this word concerns itself with the application to a progression of vortices that greatly mimics that of a wheel. This exists in the outside realm of the etheric twofold of man. There is also the chakra system, which actually originated from the great country of India and was discovered around 1500 and 500 BC. It was found in one of the country's oldest texts, the Vedas. Over time, we saw how this concept has been passed on from one generation to another, from one culture to another.

Now, do keep in mind that the chakra system is an Eastern philosophy concept. This is an important thought that will help you further comprehend what chakras are all about. You see, in most Eastern philosophies, they believed in mind-body dualism. In theory, the mind and the body are said to be distinct types of natures or substances. In fact, there are some philosophers who have shared how this implies that the mind and the body not only differ in terms of meaning but also in terms of the kind of entity they are considered to be. It was Descartes who started to ask questions, such as "Are we mind or bodies?" While we won't delve much into this particular question, we would like you to take this into account as you go about this book: the chakra system is a system that affects both aspects - the mind and the body. Even though some philosophers claim that the body is merely illusory and the mind or the spirit is considered more valued, the chakra system is very much interlaced with an individual's overall health. When you make an effort to be healthy, there is a chance that you are only treating the body or the mind, but never both. As a result, these aches and pains that you feel rarely go away for good. With the discovery of chakra meditation, which we will discuss in the suc-ceeding paragraphs, you are given a chance to treat the wellbeing of a person wholly. Because if we are to tru-ly accept man's dualistic nature, the mind is very much interlaced with the body plane, and vice versa.

What Is Chakra Meditation?

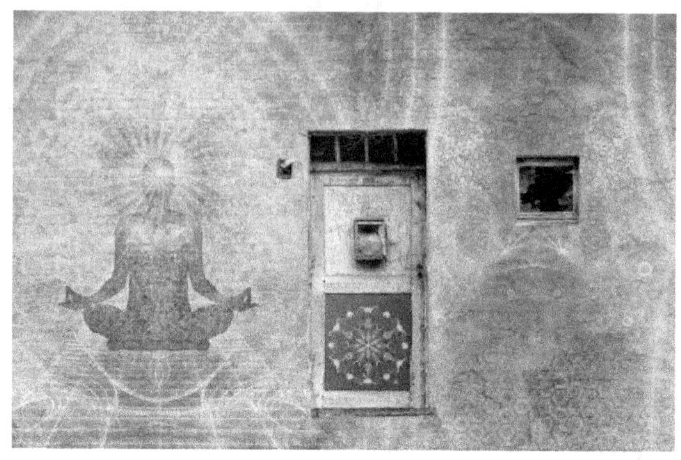

When it comes to chakra meditation, it is important to familiarize yourself with its history, as well as how people from ancient times would regard the chakra system. For them, chakras are these energy points throughout the body. It determines one's health and overall capacity. These chakra points may be the reason as to why someone may be sick. Thus, our earlier ancestors made it sure that they pay careful attention to how their chakras are well-balanced. Fast forward to today, chakras are now referenced in various modern yoga classes - even on a regular basis, but this isn't particularly new. We are simply reusing and recycling the ideas of earlier civilizations. The concept of the chakra system was passed down on to one generation from another by word of mouth. It was an oral tradition before it was ever written in books and scriptures. Nevertheless, the practice of yoga is actually based around the idea of the chakras. Both of these posits the same goal of achieving a well-balanced chakra system to keep the mind and body healthy, in other words, to achieve holistic health.

It is true that modern man will always come back to ancient philosophies, very much like this one. In fact, there are those who believed that this is a great way to manage a modern man's very demanding lives. Truly, we all live in a very fast-paced lifestyle that we often forget to take a step back and simply breathe. As a result, our holistic health is jeopardized. With a changing perspective toward the health of both our minds and bodies, people tend to return to alternative medicinal processes for a less invasive way to gain spirituality, reduce stress, and even manage our physical and emotional imbalances. On another note, it is also crucial to pay attention to what is already obvious to us in terms of our health. After reading this book, you'll soon realize that chakra meditation is basically practicing the art of being mindful. With our fast-paced lives and well-advanced technological innovations, we tend to neglect the existence of a particular matter that may already be visible to the eye. In fact, there are those who are capable of actually seeing these chakra points. This mastery is caused by years of practice and meditation. In addition, they are more equipped at identifying the reasons for why their body is acting the way it is or why their mind thinks the way it does. This part, which is often invisible to the majority of the population, is an important aspect that allows the flow of energy through our body. Without the proper flow of this energy, our body will most likely be dead. These points keep our bodies alive and our minds sane. The absence of a well-balanced chakra system can gravely affect our well-being.

The Benefits Of Each Of Your Chakras

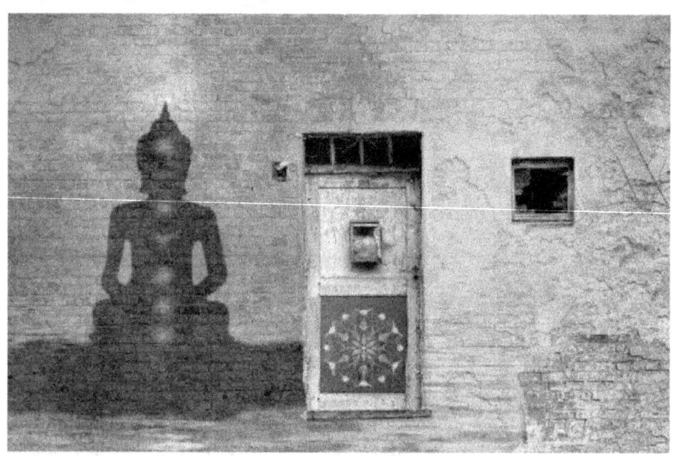

Beyond a corresponding shade and sound - one-syllable vibrations, which are referred to as Bija mantras - are said to resonate with the strength of each energy point. Nevertheless, note that the chakras have critical correspondences to a variety of principles, instincts, and emotions. There are about 114 chakra points in our body.

Chakra points that are considered as even numbers are very much associated with the female qualities, consisting of compassion, emotions, and openness. On another note, those that are considered as odd-numbered energy points correspond with masculine characteristics, such as self-control and the assertion of one's self. It is also believed that these energy points are heavily impacted by using one's inner thoughts and desires, as well as the immediate environment surrounding us. Also, keep in mind that each of these energy points is associated with a body part. As a whole, it can truly affect the entire body. The six chakras - although, we will discuss the seven basic chakras in this book - help enable excretion, reproduction, digestion, circulation, respiration, and cognition. Channels, which are also called Nadis or Meridians, connect the different energy points to one another and assist in the travel of the Prana or Chi that passes through it. Out of the 114 chakras, there are about 72,000 Nadis in our body.

In our body, there are certain imbalances affected by how our chakra system operates. This can relate to particular diseases, emotions, ailments, or even signs and symptoms of impending sickness. There are a number of educators and practitioners who specialize in this field - chakra balancing; however, there are various beginner-friendly techniques and methods that may aid and further assist you in your chakra work at home. Many herbal health shops and online retailers offer chakra-specific merchandise for color, sensory, sound, and aroma therapies. Getting used to the act of performing positive Asanas, which you may associate with various yoga poses, can also clear blocks and help you attain holistic health or prevent the overloading of your chakra points. With each chakra, we've provided

corresponding necessary oils, crystals, colors, affirmations, and healing foods that will further help you
achieve a more balanced chakra system. Nevertheless,
without further ado, here are some beginner insights on
the seven basic chakras.

- **The Root Chakra**

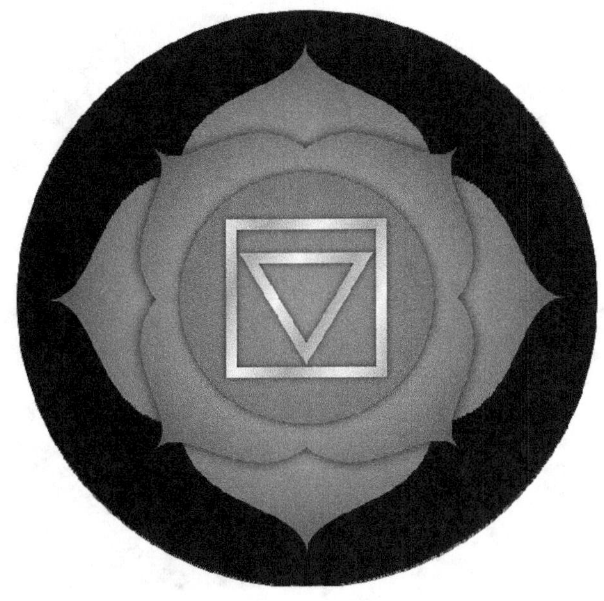

To discover this chakra, start by sitting in an Indian or Lotus position. Do remember that this particular chakra is at your tailbone. By carefully sitting in a Lotus position, you can feel your so-called "roots." Moreover, if you meditate on your root chakra, you extend your feeling of being stable and grounded. This also pertains to our bare necessities in life, such as security, shelter, and food. Many also assume of the root chakra as the place where our monetary steadiness or financial independence and stability is harnessed. This allows us to loosen up and take into account that the floor is usually underneath us. A balanced root chakra lessens our anxiety of any uncertainties that may come. Furthermore, it is also the chakra point that heavily deals with humility.

- **The Sacral Chakra**

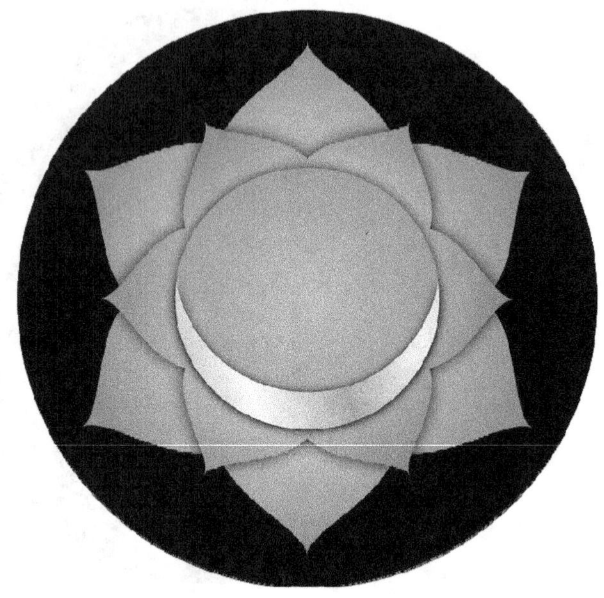

The Sacral Chakra is positioned two inches beneath and two inches inward one's umbilical cord. It is the chakra of selflessness, graciousness, and pleasure. Sacral meditation can lead humans to become more charitable. It paves the way to a healthier relationship with those around them. Furthermore, it also eliminates any emotions related to the feeling of depression, anxiety, and loneliness. Nonetheless, the sacral chakra enhances an individual's insight and intuition.

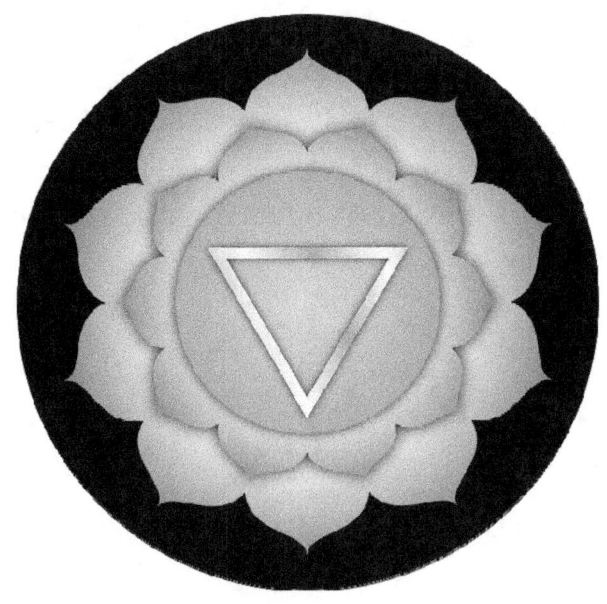

This chakra is positioned in our upper abdomen. The solar plexus chakra is described as the point where one's ability to experience self-assurance and control is harnessed. Most human beings definitely are familiar with the feeling of an unbalanced solar plexus chakra. If you have ever had the feeling of butterflies in your stomach, then it could mean that your solar plexus chakra is feeling weak or imbalanced. Oftentimes, when someone is worried or anxious, they would often put their hands on their stomach. This particular act of touching this area brings about a kind of stimulation, making the act a very subtle kind of chakra meditation. Moreover, if you ever find yourself doubting your capacities, it'll do you good to meditate on this particular chakra as it'll greatly help you with your self-esteem. This is also the reason why "butterflies in your stomach" is usually used in cases when you are talking to a crush. Deep down, you feel that you are not confident enough to strike a normal conversation; thus, you feel nervous and feel like you're not yourself. Well, those butterflies are telling you that maybe it's time to sneak in a few minutes of chakra meditation every day.

- **The Heart Chakra**

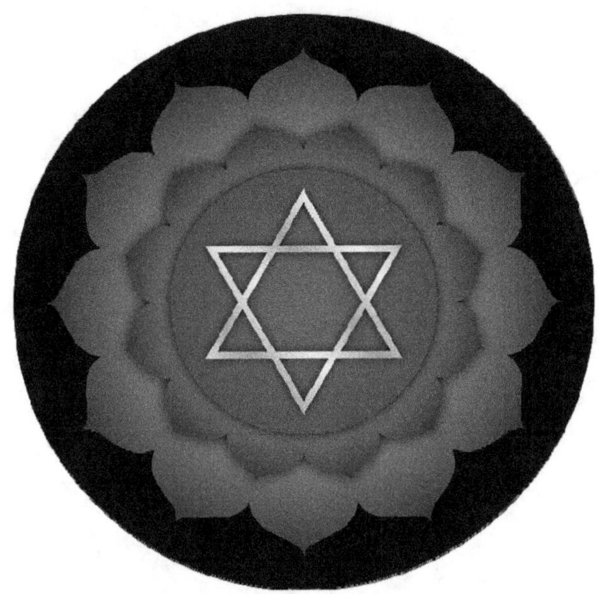

The heart chakra is located in the middle of the chest. Meditating on it can open your capacity to love others and yourselves. Also, this particular chakra allows us to experience pleasure and internal peace. There are many physical advantages to meditating on this particular chakra, some of which are as follows: it lowers our cholesterol, blood pressure, and regulates the heartbeat.

- **The Throat Chakra**

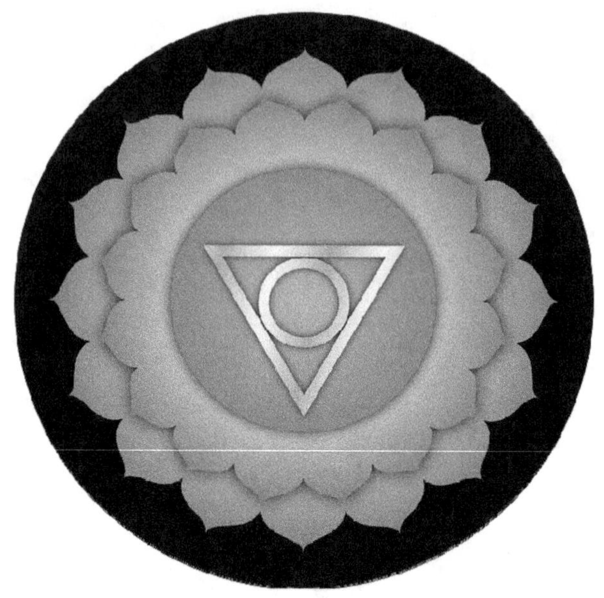

The throat chakra is located at the throat; however, it controls one's hearing as well. Nonetheless, it is deemed as the chakra of conversation and balance. Throat chakra meditation brings about the ability to clearly express what we are thinking and our capacity to listen to other people. It can be a high-quality motivator in the launch of built-up poor thoughts. Those that are considered to have wholesome throat chakras experience a state of relaxation even amidst their fears and weaknesses. For them, creativity is far greater; thus, they feel the need to hear other people's opinions and thoughts because they view this as something beneficial.

- **The Third Eye Chakra**

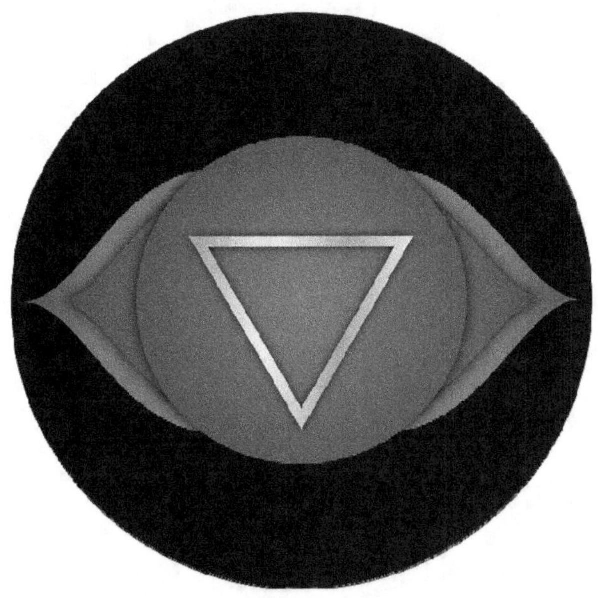

The third eye chakra is the chakra between the eyes. This is also regarded as the Brow Chakra. Third eye chakra meditation helps an individual focus and establish a mentality that regards the bigger picture rather than the minuscule details. People who often meditate in this area are relieved from overwhelming feelings because they would often see certain events as uncontrollable. Instead, they focus on the bigger picture, which is why they are less anxious if one or two things don't go according to their plan.

- **The Crown Chakra**

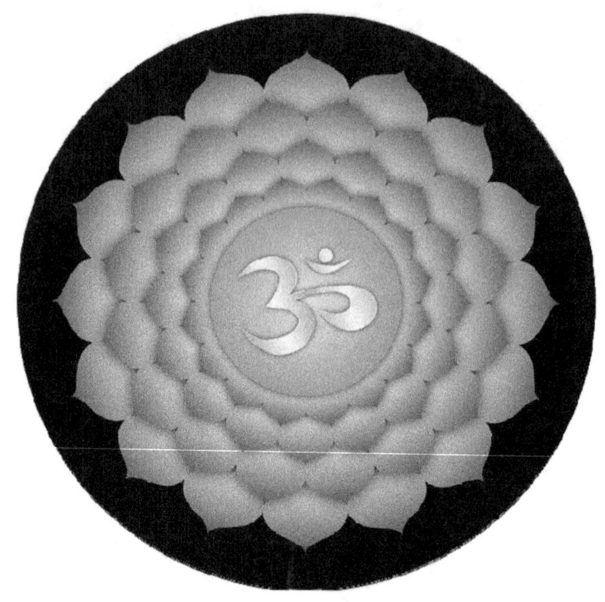

The best possible chakra sits atop of the head. It maintains the body and allows it to become familiar and associated with one's spiritual foundations. It is regularly pictured as the pinnacle of a giant oval. The bottom of which, as you already know, is the root chakra. The crown chakra is a principal entryway for the energy to enter the body. When it comes to crown chakra meditation, it is believed that it opens our minds to the holistic beauty of everything; thus, bring about one's holistic health because the individual is so in line with what the universe is providing to them. There is pure bliss and, with this targeted meditation, you can frequently experience this amazing oneness with everything around you.

It has been said that the human body was first brought into existence through the energies in the universe. There is something to be said here, that's for sure! If you are to look at it closely, people have been blinded by technological advancements over the past couple of decades that they fail to realize some of the more basic truths that our ancestors believed in. The chakra system is a framework that will allow mankind to survive longer than what is expected. Now, we know that the way mankind thinks had also evolved into using a more scientific approach. Thus, we would like to present to you the facts concerning the chakra framework with as much evidence as we can. All that we ask of you is to keep an open mind when you are reading through the succeeding chapters. Moreover, if you are already convinced that attaining a more balanced and well-maintained chakra system is what you need to be able to live a good life, then that's good. All that is left to do is to equip yourself with the necessary information and experience when it comes to meditating.

Chapter 2: Meditation 101: How To Properly Balance Your Chakras

Basic Meditation vs. Chakra Meditation vs. Mindfulness Meditation

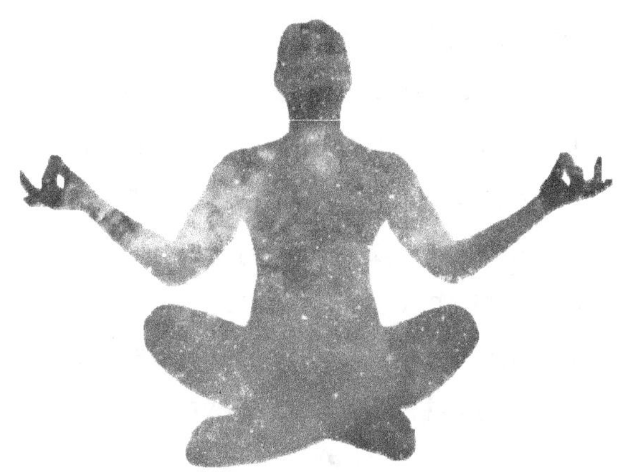

To ensure that we are all on the same page, meditation is basically the act of providing time for relaxation. It is also a time to heighten your attention. In a stressful world, it is important to listen to what our senses are telling us. Even though the 20th century is full of technological benefits, these often dull our senses. In fact, researchers have suggested that the act of meditating is more than just a temporary stress relief. Mental fitness experts, religious leaders, as well as educators have developed a number of meditation types. They suggested that there is a structure to be followed, yet you can easily alter it to suit your needs. Moreover, those who are well-acquainted with the practice of meditating is provided with an opportunity that will help enhance bodily wellbeing, as well as emotional health, because the chakra system is all about holistic health. Thus, you can rest assured that it targets both the mind and the body. However, there is no correct way to meditate or no one-size-fits-all answer to the question, "How does one meditate effectively?" This realization can only mean that humans are allowed to discover various types of meditation until they can successfully find the right one for them. With this in mind, do note that what works for others may not work for you. You see, meditation is a structure of mindfulness that encourages practitioners to live in the moment and to become more aware of their immediate surroundings, instead of dwelling on what has been or what could have been.

Mindfulness meditation is something people can do at anytime and anywhere. Let's give an example for this point to be more cohesive: while waiting in line at the grocery store, a person who is mindful may lightly observe their surroundings, consisting of the sights, sounds, and smells that they experience. The ability to become mindful of your surroundings can be achieved by following whatever type of meditation that you may follow. Breath cognizance encourages practitioners to be conscious of their breathing, whilst innovative leisure attracts the right attention to certain parts of the body that experiences anxiety. Since the art of being mindful is a frequent topic discussed in various types of meditation, it has been notably studied. Researchers have found out that this can perform the following: lessen impulsiveness, improve focus, improve memory, reduce fixation on bad emotions, enhancement of your satisfaction within a relationship, and the control over emotional reactions. There is even evidence that suggests how mindfulness might also improve health and cure sickness. A good example was when African-American individuals with chronic kidney illnesses were subjected to regular meditation. Researchers found out that mindfulness meditation can help decrease the subjects' blood pressure.

This meditation technique, which has become extremely famous in the West, is based on the teachings of Buddha. Mindfulness meditation can be instrumental in assisting you in recognizing how the mind works. This self-knowledge serves as a foundation for overcoming dissatisfaction, impatience, intolerance, and many of the different habits that keep us from achieving fuller and happier lives. Ideally, to achieve a state of mindfulness through meditation, one must combine attention with awareness. All that's required is a disciplined meditation-friendly posture and the willingness to be truthful with yourself. The best-known center of attention of mindfulness meditation is the breathing exercise; unbiased commentary of bodily sensations is another common technique. Whenever you find your ideas wandering, just simply be aware of them, and try to breathe through the process. It may sound very easy, but people have claimed that they have troubles meditating for longer than three minutes. Remember, mindfulness meditation has been proven to limit depression, stress, and anxiety. In addition, it fosters resilience, an attitude that helps you cope up with challenging situations without ever compromising your peace of mind. Basically, what you want to achieve here is the balance among all of your bodily functions, as well as that of the mind.

Now, let us dive into the nitty-gritty of chakra meditation. This is a form of meditation that helps you activate, open, and balance the seven main chakras. Moreover, it is encouraged that chakra meditation is to be practiced for about 15 to 30 minutes every session for maximum benefit. Do keep in mind that chakra meditation is harder than you think. We are not asking you to sit down in a comfortable position and simply breathe. We are asking you to become more aware of your surroundings. It takes focus and commitment. Thus, if you want to balance all of your chakra points, a certain level of expertise in chakra meditation is required. For beginners, they often practice chakra meditation with a guided recording or with a teacher.

When it comes to chakra meditation, remember to choose a focal point among the different chakra centers in the body. Seven chakras are believed to run from the bottom of the spine to the top of the head. Depending on what you want to achieve or what aspect in life you would like to target, there would be a corresponding chakra point to focus on. Each is associated with a color and corresponds to extraordinary factors of our body and mind. With enough practice, you can focus on a single chakra or on all seven of them. The goal is to stimulate and unblock every chakra point. You'll learn more about these in the succeeding chapters.

What You Need To Know About Chakra Meditation

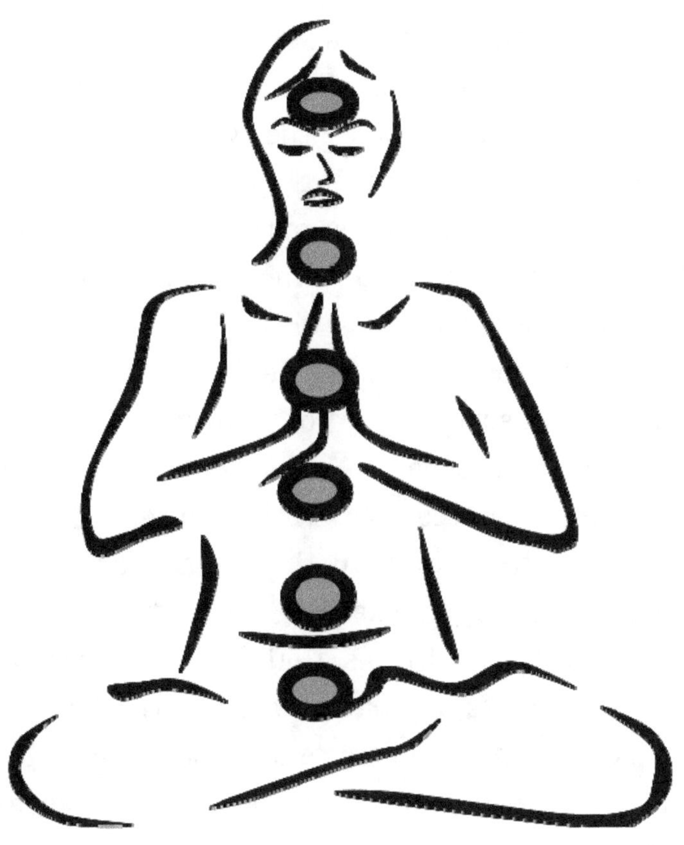

So to further understand what chakra meditation can bring to the table, it is important to first contemplate as to how huge and influential these chakra centers are. Take note that our existence - both the mind and body - is an ideal impression of our convictions, considerations, and feelings. It is the physical appearance of our internal convictions that makes us who we are or where our identity is based upon. The body and all that we experience here is a pictorial portrayal of what we accept to be valid about ourselves. The vast majority of these convictions are in an oblivious state. The chakra points resemble fiery engines inside our body's psychological and physical energy field. Each chakra point is identified with an alternate part of our lives. As explained, the wellbeing of a chakra is administered by our convictions about ourselves. For example, the root chakra is often identified with our feeling of association with other people, which may be related to our sense of survival. In the event that an individual realizes that someone is considered as hazardous or troublesome, the root chakra - through one's awareness and mindfulness - will alert the individual that it would be better to avoid further developing a relationship with the said hazardous or troublesome person. Let's give an example so that you are better able to understand this situation: an abused person will most likely stay or return to their abuser because they are not mindful or aware of the damage the other person is bringing them. As a result, the abused continuously welcomes their abuser into their life with the belief that they are good for them or the other way around. Through the powers of root chakra meditation, there is a possibility that the abused will become more grounded with reality. On another note, the third eye chakra can also assist the root chakra in helping the individual see the bigger picture - the truth that they are a victim of abuse.

Do consider that the seven main chakras are a piece of the most ordinarily known framework of our energy points, which as you may have already known, is situated along the spine up to the very top of our heads. Moreover, this standard chakra framework depends on a Hindu chakra framework that perceives seven unmistakable "wheels" or "focuses" of energy that are ceaselessly moving along the human body's spinal section. With each having its very own shading and vibrational recurrence, these wheels are the impetuses of cognizance and human capacity. They oversee different intense subject matters, from our survival impulses and confidence to our capacity to convey and experience love.

Before we proceed to explain the seven basic chakras, their purpose, and what they can contribute to our lives, we would like to give you a rundown on what you can expect from this chapter, as well as the succeeding chapters. We have attempted to make all of the details presented in this book as cohesive as possible. Thus, most of the corresponding data - particularly, those associated with the seven main chakras - will be repeated more than once. We would like you to get the idea that all of these are actually interconnected. There is a sense of oneness in all of these and you must be able to look at the bigger picture. Yes, each of the seven main chakras can provide you with a particular list of benefits, but there is more to it when you truly start aiming for a much higher goal - that is achieving ultimate enlightenment by balancing all of the seven chakras. This means that you have started from the bottom, which is the root chakra, and have made your way up to the very top that is the crown chakra, opening it up so that the universe can provide you with the wisdom that you need to attain holistic health; thus, a happy life! Don't worry, we will be explaining this concept and process as you read along with the following chapters. With all of these in mind, here are some of the basic information on the seven main chakras.

How To Effectively Awaken Your Seven Chakras

- **The Root Chakra**

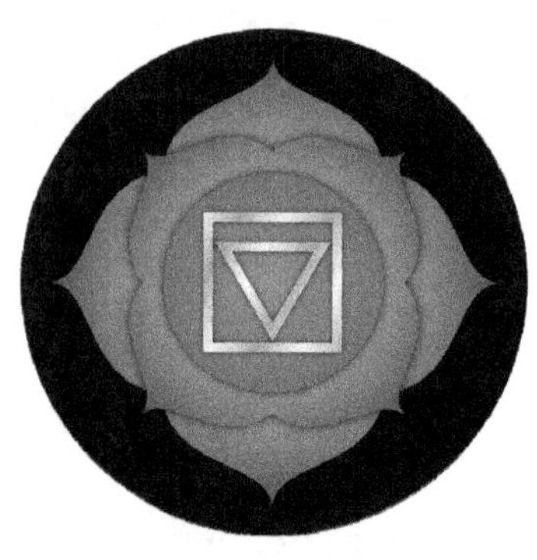

The root chakra, being the first chakra, is the most physical one. This implies that any action that makes one progressively mindful of the body will reinforce this energy point. This specifically pertains to our physical movement in the world that we live in. One can do sports, combative techniques, strolling, yoga, and Taichi, yet each of this action can make a difference as to how we live our lives. Moreover, this also pertains to some of the more ordinary actions like housekeeping, dishwashing, and vehicle cleaning. It is significant not to do things that make one suffer and to not try too hard or exert too much force on a particular action. Fatigue is simply not great and it can affect both the mind and the body of an individual. The root chakra is about associating yourself with the ground. Sayings like "Keep your eyes on the stars, but your feet on the ground" pass on a decent message that pertains to our ability to strive for excellence, yet be humble at the same time.

Nevertheless, if you want to truly awaken your root chakra, follow these simple steps: you must start with a standing position. Be sure to stand upright with your feet apart and make sure that you are not tensed. Somewhat twist your knees and put your pelvis fairly forward. Keep your body flexible and ensure that your weight is uniformly disseminated over the soles of your feet. Hold this position for a few minutes. By focusing on the muscles that are between your rear-end, the root chakra is invigorated. Every time you breathe in, contract these muscles internally and, when you breath out, release the muscles. Repeat this process step for a few minutes.

The best part about this is that it can be done while sitting down, standing up, or when you're walking around. Moreover, you can also chant a particular mantra to help you with the process. You'll learn more about mantras in the succeeding chapters.

- **The Sacral Chakra**

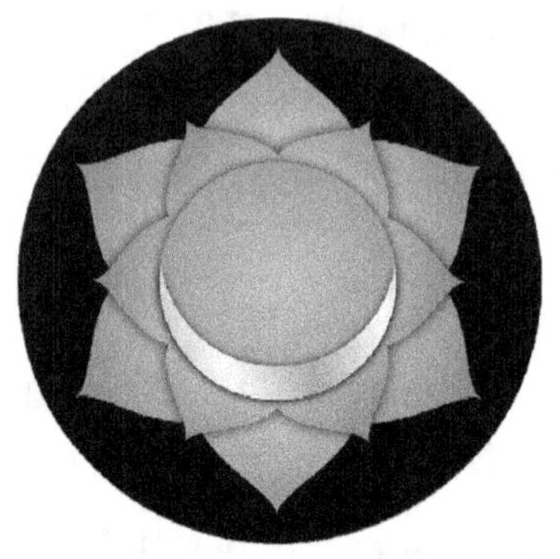

Did you, at any point in time, ever met someone who transmits a kind, warm, and positive aura? The sort of individual who grasps the world and with whom you promptly feel great and calm? All things considered, odds say that you have met somebody whose second chakra is well-adjusted. Individuals with a decent sacral chakra, or Swadhisthana chakra, are more in touch with their general surroundings. They are lively, genuinely steady, and caring that anyone who meets them would experience a genuine euphoria throughout their day.

The Swadhisthana chakra is the focal point of enthusiasm, positive feeling, delight, and inventiveness. This chakra is situated in the pelvic zone, around four fingers below where your stomach is. At the point when Swadhisthana chakra is out of equalization, you may experience trust issues, carry on cold and inaccessible relationships with others, or you may encounter the inverse and be excessively subordinate over the power others have on you. Individuals with sacral chakra imbalances regularly feel overpowered and extremely touchy as they often experience sexual issues. They are inclined to experience the ill effects of addictions and they appear to be attracted to strife and dramatization. Imbalances of the second chakra additionally show itself on a physical level through urinary issues, kidney issues, gynecological issues, and lower back pains.

As most yoga professionals know, feelings and strains will develop in the pelvic region. That clarifies why there is such a large number of hip opening stances in yoga. On the off chance that you are not persuaded of the legitimacy of this statement, give it a shot for yourself and watch the distinction in adaptability in your hip joints on days when you feel loose and optimistic, as well as on days when you feel enthusiastic and focused. It is likely that your adaptability has decreased essentially when you are in a passionate perspective. By including some hip-opening activities in your yoga practice, you don't just relinquish physical strain, yet you also discharge enthusiastic blockages, subsequently invigorating and adjusting your sacral chakra. Additionally, adjusting postures, such as the Kakasana or the Crow Pose, as well as standing stances like the Trikonasana or the Triangle Pose are productive stances to adjust an individual's Swadhisthana chakra.

On another note, one of the more typical reasons for a blocked or overactive Sacral chakra is psychological weight. When you are not ready to relinquish feelings, be it dread, outrage, disappointment, or disgrace, these negative feelings develop until they structure a substantial block pulling you down rationally and physically. As an outcome, the enthusiasm you get from your second chakra may close itself totally as a means to assure itself, or despite what might be expected, it may end up becoming over dynamic, bringing about outrageous emotional episodes, melancholy, and so on.

Nevertheless, there are various approaches to discharge these negative feelings. A good and basic example would be to talk about it as it slowly allows yourself to acknowledge the existence of these feelings. You can either talk to someone about it or you can simply write it down on a diary or journal. Moreover, you can also perform certain activities that allow you to express yourself, such as dancing, singing, painting, and more. As explained, there is no one-size-fits-all answer as to how you should meditate. There are so many approaches to follow that you simply need to find the right one which will work for you. It's really astounding how much alleviation you may feel once you have figured out how to express and relinquish blocked or stifled feelings.

If you are at a loss as to how you can awaken or balance your second chakra, start by putting your hands in your lap, palms up, over one another. Your left hand should be placed underneath your right hand and the palms should be in contact with the back of the fingers of your right hand. The tips of the thumbs should be aligned delicately. As you meditate, focus on your sacral chakra, which is situated on your lower back, and try to chant words of encouragement.

- ## The Solar Plexus Chakra

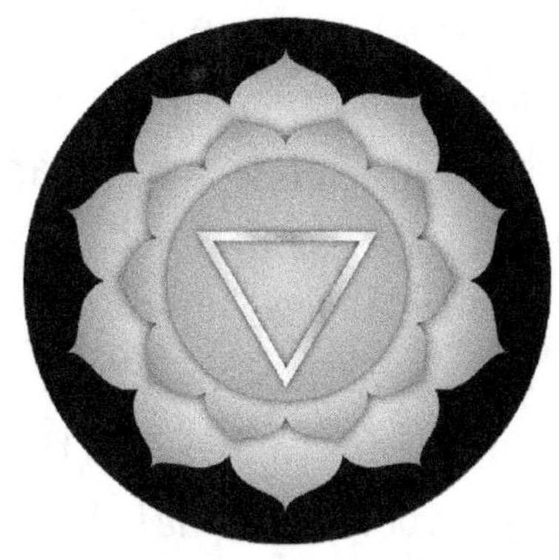

The solar plexus chakra or Manipura chakra is regularly alluded to as the chakra of individual power. This is found over the navel at the base of our rib cage. Moreover, it is also regarded as the seat of our inner self and where we attract inspiration to accomplish our objectives. It administers our capacity to accomplish the objectives we set for ourselves, directs our confidence, and regulates our crude feelings as we draw on it for our self-control. Since this chakra is situated close to the mid-region of our body, it influences numerous inner organs, such as the kidneys, digestive organs, and pancreas. Stomach ulcers and conceivable weight issues can likewise be credited to a lopsided solar plexus. What's more, we may experience the ill effects of back issues, torpidity and, in light of the fact that this chakra is associated with our feeling of sight, we may encounter fogginess with our vision.

Note that physical diseases dramatically affect our sense of passion and otherworldly state and, on the off chance that we focus on these energies inside our bodies, we could assume responsibility for the ailments we feel that are unleashing destruction on our bodies. Also, we may feel frail or ineffectual, which can prompt negative musings and misery. At times, we will question ourselves and our achievements or even doubt our loved ones. Nervousness and low self-esteem frequently go hand-in-hand with an imbalanced solar plexus. However, if we are able to successfully achieve a balanced solar plexus, our point of view improves, reactions and issues are simpler to deal with, and you may have complete command over your feelings and opinions over certain things. The sense of self is simpler to deal with. You will comprehend and acknowledge your internal harmony and transmit that acknowledgment outward, coming to acknowledge individuals and the things around you. Whenever adjusted, our solar plexus gives us trust in ourselves and our exhibition of certain tasks. We feel confident and pleased with our work at accomplishing our objectives. The solar plexus chakra is associated with the sense of sight. It is said that astigmatic individuals may have an excess feeling of dread or frailty, while those who are far-sighted may hold indignation or blame.

We can draw on our own capacity to help invigorate this particular chakra. Practicing our self-control carries us closer to our objectives, yet reinforces our chakra and enables us to process the more troublesome circumstances and pessimism in our lives. Moreover, there have been attempts at balancing this particular chakra. Again, it is best to experiment with various types of meditation so that you are better able to find the right one for you. Nevertheless, most beginners would start with activities that break the dullness of a routinary life. You can enroll in a class and start a new hobby. You can also volunteer or simply learn new things every day by reading books. Routinary schedules will sustain our sentiments of frailty. Break the dull idleness of your life and have a go at something new. Venture outside of your everyday practice and go adventuring, regardless of whether that implies heading off to a new mall that recently opened up in your neighborhood or you would try a peculiar dish at a new restaurant. Indeed, even little breaks in routine will imbue you with vitality and imperativeness. One little change can give you the inspiration and reestablished vitality that you need.

- **The Heart Chakra**

Situated in the focal point of the chest, the heart

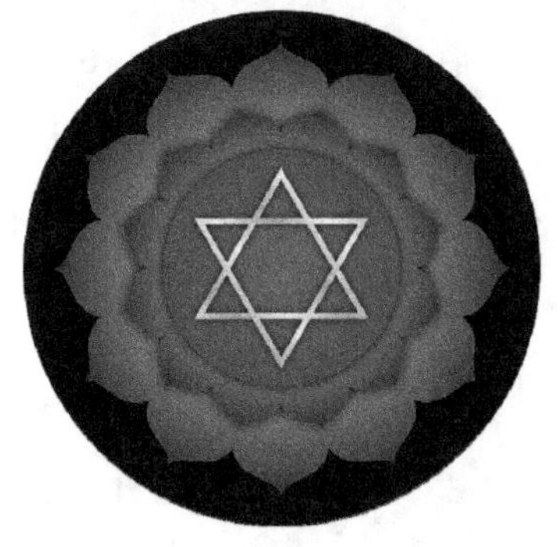

chakra does not only pertain to the heart. It is also associated with the lungs, thymus organ, and cardiovascular system. In Sanskrit, this chakra is called Anahata. Truth be told, it is the profound spot where past encounters and complaints can never hurt us again. The Anahata chakra is related to the color green, which speaks to change. Those with an open and all-around adjusted heart chakra are loaded with affection, absolution, and empathy. In any case, if this chakra is blocked, outrage, melancholy, contempt, and envy will most likely show.

Figuring out how to open the heart chakra may be a challenge but it is certainly not impossible. Regardless of whether an individual has encountered blockage in this chakra point since adolescence, or because of one's ongoing grief, opening the heart is the beginning of your process of recuperation and self-healing. Note that there are various things that can cause a vigorous blockage in this chakra point. Some of these may include several ailments, stress, and a clash between opposing forces. At the point when your Anahata chakra point is blocked, it can negatively affect your physical and passionate wellbeing. In the body, this can interpret as poor course and circulatory strain limits. The heart and lungs are altogether affected extraordinarily by the Anahata chakra. Profoundly, a blocked fourth chakra can cause a sense of detachment among other people, an absence of sympathy, and powerlessness to confide in oneself or others. Profound uncertainty and fears are likewise normal. However, when these are left unchecked, these can further develop into manipulative practices.

Reflection can reestablish appropriate vitality stream to the heart chakra. What's more, since reflection is such a profound activity that is close to home involvement, you should set aside an effort to discover a training that works best for you. Here are a couple of contemplation tips for to regain balance to your heart chakra: sit or lie in a place that doesn't strain your spine or joints; discover a spot where you are relaxed and would not require too much effort; make a habit to wear clothes that bring about joy and happiness, probably those of the color yellow or green. Since the heart chakra usually corresponds to the color green, you can add green not only to your wardrobe but also try to surround yourself with plants as they are an incredible method to bring life into your workspace. Mantras are an extraordinary method to certify your reflection endeavors. These are not only straightforward, but they also help you achieve clarity. The mantra for the Anahata is "Yum" or "Yam." Repeat this word as you meditate, while picturing yourself opening up to the feeling of genuine love and sympathy. Mantras can be rehashed vocally or sub-vocally while you contemplate. Positive insistences can enable you to build positive vitality related to the fourth chakra. These can incorporate little notes you leave for yourself on the restroom mirror or on your work desk.

Music talks profoundly to the human soul. Uplift and draw out your reflective endeavors by consolidating music into your training. Moreover, tuning in to happy and blissful music is a helpful method to develop an inspirational point of view. Open your heart to the message of the music and enable its actual significance to reverberate profoundly inside of you. Since the heart chakra is the highlight of all seven chakras, it's where the physical and otherworldly planes meet, and the majority of this lays on an establishment of adoration and appreciation. This is actually the reason as to why it is significant for everybody to recuperate and develop their fourth chakra.

In some cases, self-contemplation can fizzle. It neglects to give you the outcomes you're anticipating. In such a situation, deciding on following a guided reflection is your best bet. In a guided reflection session, you adhere to the guidelines of a prepared meditative expert who encourages you to focus your thoughts and energy towards your Anahata chakra point.

On another note, there are other practices that best help you balance this particular chakra point. All you need to remember is that love heightens when it is shared. Thus, even the simplest act can help you achieve balance with your heart chakra. Give your pets some warmth; never let a chance to display affection go to waste; do philanthropy work; attempt to comprehend the furious mental skirmishes of individuals who you meet every day. Individuals consistently leave signs when they're discouraged. Their dismal articulations simply give them away. At whatever point you feel like somebody near you is experiencing a hard time, don't simply evade them. Instead, converse with them and tune in to what they need to state. Don' t be afraid to listen to them. Also, offer them the chance to share their problems with you without fear of judgment. These little deeds of graciousness can be very helpful in balancing your Anahata chakra.

- ## The Throat Chakra

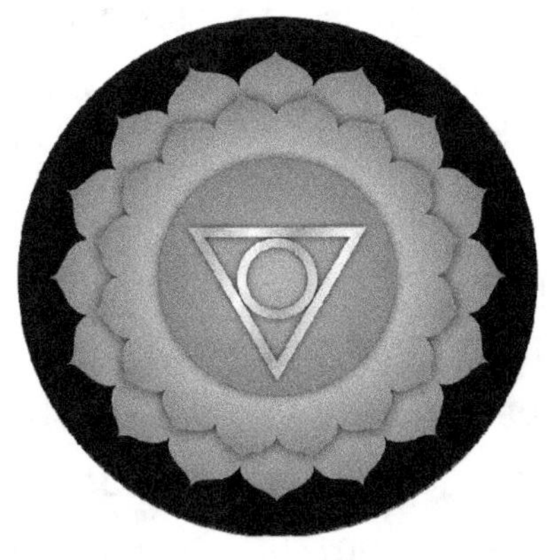

The throat chakra is simply the energy point related to articulation and correspondence. Situated at the foundation or bottom of the throat, the fifth chakra is likewise considered the source of our everyday feelings and emotions. Known as the Vishuddha chakra, it administers all zones of the mouth, jaw, throat, and thyroid organ. At the point when the throat chakra is imbalanced, you may experience dryness among certain body parts, sore throat, thyroid issues, laryngitis, and neck pains. Moreover, you may also experience melancholy, powerlessness to communicate, tension, animosity, and absence of confidence.

Signs and manifestations of an imbalanced throat chakra incorporate unreasonable talking, self-importance, deceptive nature, tentativeness, dread, and manipulative conduct. While an individual with a well-balanced throat chakra can convey what needs to be conveyed. This chakra is simply the seat of articulation and can be seen as a junction of the heart and the head - filling in as a middle person among feelings and considerations. On the off chance that you lack the capacity and trust in communicating your sentiments, thoughts, and considerations, there is a chance that you may have trouble with your throat chakra. Moreover, on the off chance that your fifth chakra is blocked, you likely experience dissatisfaction with regards to communicating your emotions. This regularly implies not having the option to locate the right words, especially when you are terrified of losing a person or thing. There may even come a time when you need to lie to yourself or other people just so that you can get what you want. Insufficiencies in the fifth chakra regularly add to various physical illnesses that can incorporate hearing issues, tonsillitis, mouth ulcers, tinnitus, bronchitis, asthma, and ear diseases.

The following are a few tips to opening your throat chakra and reestablishing harmony within one's self: it is important to learn how to listen to your inner thoughts so that you are better able to articulate them, The act of keeping quiet, which in Sanskrit is known as Mouna, is a ground-breaking exercise that can assist you with conserving, cleansing, and fortifying the vitality of your Vishuddha chakra or the extension between your heart and psyche. By rehearsing the Mouna Meditation daily, you will start, through a procedure of self-examination, to ensure that your words correspond with your actions. To guarantee that your words and actions stay tuned in to your musings, it is highly recommended to practice silence so that you can effectively concentrate on your internal thoughts and reflect. In doing so, it is best that you pick a time of the day when you don't need to interact with other people. As you meditate, don't forget some of the basic breathing exercises. On another note, listening to calming music is always a good idea. Sooner than later, you'll start to see yourself adapting to the commotion around you. You'll realize that you are slowly becoming more mindful of every detail in your surroundings. As a result, your thoughts become more at peace and organized, which will allow you to articulate them better.

- **The Third Eye Chakra**

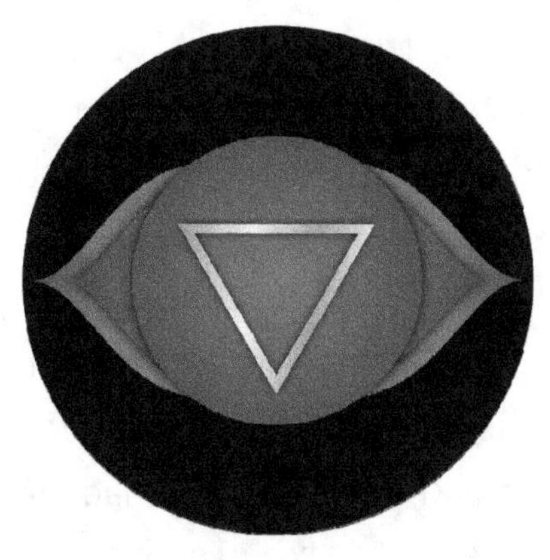

Ever thought about how to open your third eye, a.k.a. the home of your intuition? Most of the time, people would associate the third eye with "the space in the middle of," as they often hear stories about people with an open third eye that can experience mystic and spiritual happenings. Some would even claim that an open third eye allows an individual to see into the domain of the imperceptible. To have the ability to access the voice of your third eye can bring about so many benefits. For one, you'll be able to see the murmur of its insight. In the event that your unconscious is pretty boisterous, you may miss its primary message.

There are a number of ways to develop your instinct. It is the fundamental seat of discernment, as well as having the power that will allow us to see the unseen, there are those that are skeptic about the practices of opening this particular chakra point. Nevertheless, these generally exclusive practices will show up progressively in your everyday lives and you will simply garner trust in your own capabilities once you are able to balance your third eye chakra successfully. To be honest, one of the challenges as to why you may be having trouble with this chakra point is because you refuse to "open your eyes" to the possibility and grandeur of it all. Make sure that your mind is active and open to the power of the third eye chakra, and you may even find yourself surprised and amazed on the day you awaken this chakra point.

As you may have already known, there are chakra color tests that bind different various shades to the seven main chakras. For the third eye chakra, the key shading is purple. This gives you valuable data to discovering third eye chakra stones to work with. The idea is that you can discover gems including purple stones and wear them whenever you have to unblock the third eye chakra. You can likewise buy precious stones that will sit in your pocket or in the palm of your hand, enabling you to press them when you have to keep your third eye chakra open. The absolute best third eye chakra stones are as follows:

- o Purple fluorite: This semi-valuable jewel should elevate honed instinct and clear up jumbled musings. It's a perfect third eye chakra gem when you're attempting to settle on a troublesome decision and need to dispose of unessential diversions.

- o Amethyst: A popular and delightful valuable stone, amethyst is generally associated with third eye cerebral pain alleviation just as all types of meditation. A few people additionally use it to speak to astuteness.

- o Dark Obsidian: Another prominent gem from the long list of third eye precious stones. Dark obsidian advances balance among feeling and reason.

Reflection may be one of the principal things that rung a bell when you think about the inquiry "What is a chakra?". Nonetheless, third eye meditation is only one of the numerous approaches to deal with opening this chakra. Furthermore, there are a lot of chakra reflection systems for both beginner and advanced learners. On the off chance that you are starting out, this may be a good place to start; sit comfortably and close your eyes. Breathe in and breathe out multiple times, gradually and profoundly. Concentrate on the area of the third eye chakra and envision a violet circle of vitality in your temple. Keep in mind, purple is the third eye chakra's shading so it is important to picture the color clearly in your mind. As you keep on breathing in and out, picture the purple chunk of vitality getting bigger and more intense. As it does, envision it cleansing cynicism from your body. Enable yourself to feel it everywhere. Then, open your eyes when you are ready.

As you may have speculated, yoga can likewise be useful when figuring out how to adjust your chakras. In addition, keep in mind that all-natural products, vegetables, solid fats, and wholegrain nourishments will in general advance transparency all through the chakra framework. Be that as it may, there are explicit third eye chakra nourishments, and adding them to your everyday diet can forestall or battle blockages. Remember the accompanying:

o Dark Chocolate: If you like dark chocolate, don't hesitate to have as much as you need when you're attempting to open the third eye. It is said to help improve mental clearness and lift fixation. It has a great amount of magnesium, which can help you relieve yourself of stress. As a little something extra, it advances the arrival of serotonin, placing you in an increasingly positive mindset.

o Purple-Colored Food: Given that purple is the third eye's shading, every single purple nourishment advances its equalization of this chakra

point. The absolute best models incorporate eggplant, purple cabbage, red grapes, blueberries,
and blackberries.

o Omega-3: Foods that are wealthy in omega-3 can
upgrade intellectual capacity and accordingly
help to keep your third eye chakra open. Great
decisions incorporate pecans, salmon, chia seeds,
and sardines.

Lastly, we would like you to know that one of the ene-
mies of a well-balanced third eye chakra is worry and
overthinking. Thus, the most basic practice you can do
to combat this is self-care. Listen to your body and
take care of it. This includes eating a healthy diet,
getting a restful night's sleep, and exercising.

- **The Crown Chakra**

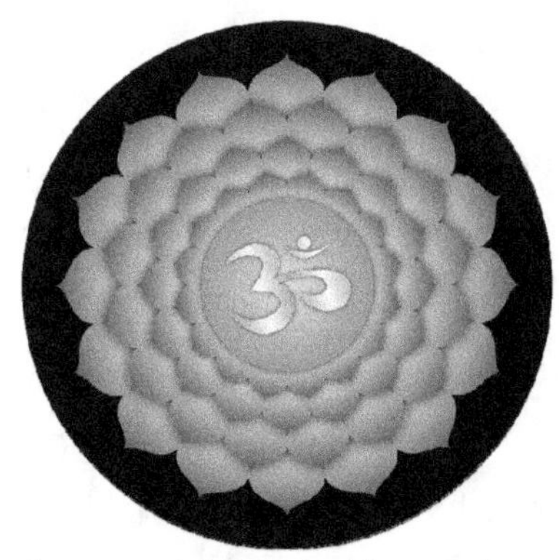

The Sahasrara chakra, also
known as the crown chakra, is
situated on the highest point
of the head. It administers internal correspondence with our
profound self. It takes into
account our relationship with
the Universal Life Force, which
is scattered through each of the seven chakras. It is
the focal point of information and edification, as well
as one's ability to express the advancement and devel-

opment of the soul all throughout our lifetime. Moreover, the crown chakra is a significant chakra that helps the other six chakras remain open. Thus, it is important to work your way from bottom to top when trying to achieve a well-balanced chakra framework. Your root chakra should be well-established before you move on to the next one because you would need to establish the ground in which you stand first. Be certain to work through all your chakras, starting with the root chakra and moving towards the crown chakra to help invigorate vitality stream and congruity. The crown chakra is the center for trust, commitment, motivation, bliss, and inspiration. It's also the center for more profound relationships with ourselves and with the power and beauty, which is actually more noteworthy than ourselves.

Consequently, it tends to be very helpful to have instruments to open the crown chakra. Here are three of our top choices that will have this chakra open in the blink of an eye!

o One approach to open the crown chakra is through motivation. For instance, think about a music show that you visited or a family gathering that you enjoyed when you were young. Keep in mind how that memory affected you. In the event that you have felt delighted and utmost happiness at how you recalled that particular memory, this could mean that your crown chakra is at work as the memory propels you to experience optimism and gratitude.

o To open the crown chakra, you can also go for a stroll at the park or read an inspiring sonnet. Anything that brings you motivation to yourself will open your crown chakra. Pause and appreciate everything that life has to offer you and consider what brings you motivation. By doing this, not only are you trying to invite positivity into your life, but you are also on your way to achieving a well-balanced crown chakra.

o The third method is through perception. Pause for a minute and picture a brilliant circle of light filling the highest point of your head. See this brilliant sphere of light developing and growing. Envision it is hoisting your contemplations and filling you with a sentiment of energy. Envision surges of brilliant light originating from the highest point of your head. Feel an open and extended inclination at the highest point of your head, as well as acknowledge your unity and solidarity with all of life. Imagine this light, which is the power of life, becoming more and more prominent than yourself. Moreover, you can also chant words of enlightenment, such as "I am associated with the power of life more noteworthy than myself." Truly feel the warmth of this light and tell yourself that you are never alone.

As you hold onto this vision, you are slowly opening the crown chakra and fortifying your association with the power of life.

As should be obvious, figuring out how to open your crown chakra is a truly important step. You will need to work with certain tools and instruments daily so as to feel more motivated, more trustworthy, and more energetic at your association with the power of life. While quietness is the most dominant and significant approach to opening the seventh chakra, there are other different practices that may help you in this process.

There are two Pranayama breathing methods you can do before reflection. You can utilize the Nadi Shodhana, or interchanging your breathing through your nostrils, and Kapalabhati, or the Skull Shining Breath.

o   Nadi Shodhanana

Nadi Shodhanana, also called the Alternate Nostril Breathing, is an amazing breathing practice with a wide array of advantages. Nadi is a Sanskrit word signifying "channel" or "stream," and Shodhana signifies "filtration." Therefore, Nadi Shodhana is basically used for clearing and filtering the unobtrusive channels of the mind and body, while at the same time adjusting its male and female perspectives. To do this, you must first start with an open sitting position - either leg over leg on the floor with a pad or mat to help with the spine, or in a seat with your feet leveled evenly on the floor. Enable the spine to protract so that the back, neck, and head are erect all through this meditative practice. Then, close the eyes.

Start by taking a full and profound inward breath followed by a moderate and more delicate exhalation. Along these lines, practice a few rounds to help stir the Prana Maya Kosha or the Vital Sheath. Then, start to overlap the tips of your forefinger and middle finger until they are in contact with the palm at the base of the thumb; this is known as the Vishnu Mudra. You will, on the other hand, utilize the thumb so that it will close the right nostril. Moreover, both the pinky and ring fingers - together - will close the left nostril. Remember, to utilize the right thumb to close your right nostril and not the other way around. Breathe out slowly but all the way through your left nostril first. Keeping the right nostril shut. If you breathe in, you're going to do it through the left nostril and let the air enter your body into your lungs. As you breathe in, enable the breath to travel upward along the other half of your body.

You will need to repeat this step but, this time, you will utilize the ring and pinky fingers of the right hand to delicately close the left nostril and exhale through the right nostril. Keeping the left nostril shut, breathe in through the right nostril, enabling the air to go up the right side of your body. This finishes one round of Nadi Shodhana. A similar example proceeds each round: breathe in through the left nostril, breathe out through the right nostril, breathe in through the right nostril, and breathe out through the left nostril. Rehash this exchanging design for a few additional rounds, concentrating your mindfulness on the pathway of the breath - up one side of the body, from the pelvic area to the top of the head, and withdrawing the air at the opposite side of your body, from the crown of the head to the pelvic area. Keep your breathing moderate all throughout the training. When you are prepared to close your training, finish your last round of Nadi Shodhana with a big exhale through your left nostril. Loosen up your correct hand and place it gently on your lap as you take a few full Yogic Breaths. Then, allow your breathing to come back to normal. As you do, assess your sense of perspective. How are you feeling? What sensations are available in your body? Carefully watch how this exercise impacted you. At some point, delicately open your eyes when you are ready, proceeding to concentrate a portion of your mindfulness internally. Gradually get up and go about your chores for the remainder of your day.

There are numerous varieties of Nadi Shodhana. Some further developed other procedures to fuse breathing maintenance. The above guidelines are simply intended to give you an appropriate prologue to Nadi Shodhana. Obviously, it is in every case best to become familiar with other strategies from a certified instructor.

o Kapalabhati Pranayama

Kapalabhati - or Kapalbhati - Pranayama is considered as an advanced breathing technique that brings about the cleansing of one' s lungs, respiratory system, and sinuses. Furthermore, the practice of this particular breathing technique can prevent illnesses and allergies. It can increase one' s supply of oxygen in the body. Most importantly, it energizes and stimulates the brain as it prepares everything else for meditation, considering the fact that this exercise would require the individual high level of focus. With that in mind, practicing the Kapalabhati Pranayama before every meditation can increase your chance of becoming more mindful.

On another note, we would like to warn anyone who decides to perform this breathing technique. Since this is an advanced breathing exercise, it is important to acquaint yourself first with the basic Pranayamas, such as the Ocean Breath (Ujjayi Pranayama) and the Three-Part Breath (Dirga Pranayama). Also, do not practice this is you are known to experience high blood pressure, hernia, or heart disease. Women who are pregnant and those who have respiratory problems, such as emphysema or asthma, are also advise to not use this approach.

Nevertheless, if you are well-equipped and knowledgeable about the basic Pranayamas and are considered to be healthy enough to perform this breathing exercise, then go ahead and start by sitting in a comfortable position. Do note that your spine should be straight and your abdomen must not be compressed. There are various seating positions that you may want to try: you can use the upright seated position, also known as the Easy Pose (Sukhasana), or the Hero Pose (Virasana) where you sit on your heels while your shins are tucked beneath your thighs and your knees are bent, or you can simply sit on a chair. If you do sit on a chair, be sure that your feet are flat on the floor. Then, your hands must be placed on your knees with your palms facing down. Start to concentrate on your lower belly. A good technique to bring awareness to this area is to place your hands on top of each other on your belly, rather than on your knees. Of course, this is only optional. You can bring awareness to your lower belly without having to touch it. Next, deeply inhale through your nostrils as your contract your lower belly. As you release the contraction, exhale deeply. Start slowly, but proceed to aim for about 65 to 70 contractions every minute. Remember, always go at it on your own pace. If you, at any point during this exercise feel dizzy, stop and take a rest. You can repeat the Kapalabhati Pranayama as many times as you want, depending on your level of expertise. The key here is to never force yourself to do something that would eventually hurt you.

What You Need To Know About Your Third Eye

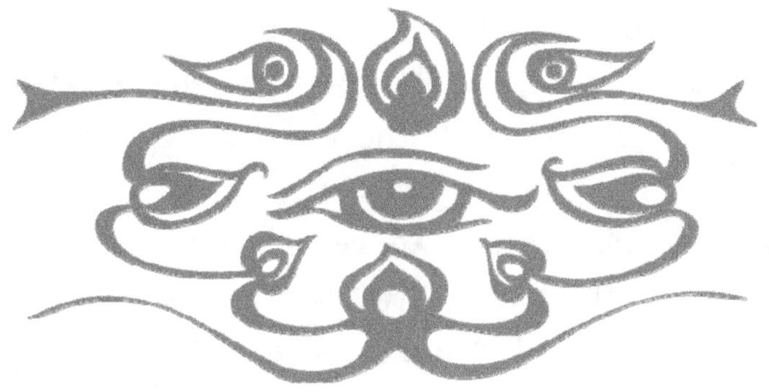

The third eye chakra is the 6th of the seven primary chakras - which means it's related with the color purple, the second-to-the-last shading in the rainbow, and that it's one of our most significant wellsprings of otherworldliness. The third eye chakra interfaces oneself and the world, enabling us to rise above duality.

It is situated between the eyebrows, simply over the scaffold of the nose, and not in the focal point of the temple, which is a typical misinterpretation in many unreliable sources. The third eye chakra is additionally called the Ajna chakra, which means "order" or "seeing," indicating that this is responsible for how we see the world around us. While it is prevalently about otherworldliness and the supernatural, the third eye chakra is additionally connected with the eyes, ears, pituitary organ, pineal organ, and sensory system.

With its area between the eyes, the third eye chakra identifies with one's vision, yet it goes a lot further than exacting visual perception. This chakra administers our discernment, instinct, and understanding, and allows us to see both the physical and the spiritual realm. At the point when the third eye chakra is open, we consider things to be what they are and accurately intuit the things we can't see. In any case, when this chakra is blocked or unbalanced, we will disregard our instincts and neglect to see what is really happening in front of us. On the off chance that the third eye winds up blocked, you may likewise end up getting progressively connected to results and being either excessively legitimate or excessively enthusiastic. Individuals with a blockage in the third eye chakra oftentimes experience discouragement, tension, and a heightened level of suspicion. Physically, it can prompt cerebral pains, vision issues, sinus inconvenience, and hypertension.

The third eye chakra opens normally, yet the procedure is slow and you can't hope to have your third eye blooming after a couple of reflections. The initial move towards lighting the fire inside this chakra is to have more time with yourself and measure the significance of otherworldliness in your life. Our third eye is a piece of our lively body, it has been with us since the very birth of this physical body that has been given to us, and it has consistently been actuated and turning. As kids, even before our mind changes to the condition of adapted beings, we're only glad to be alive, glad to encounter all that life brings to the table. It's exceptionally regular for the cutting edge individual to arrive at early adulthood with a sense of discouragement, tension, and dread about existence, one's self, and what's to come. The period from age six to 20 is so serious and overpowering that we totally lose ourselves in the hallucination of realism and vanity.

It's not hard to discover guided reflections that put emphasis on the third eye chakra; actually, a few customs instruct that the consideration ought to consistently be on the third eye during contemplation. To unblock this chakra with meditation, envision a dark blue-purple ball of energy at the third eye, and see it getting greater and more intense. As it does, feel as if your whole body is being enveloped with the energy of the third eye. You may always want to repeat certain attestations, either on your mind or out loud, so that you are better able to remove any obstructions that may be preventing you from opening your third eye. You can say "I am in contact with my internal direction," "I tune in to my most profound astuteness," or "I confide in my instincts." These are the absolute best insistences since they remind us to let our third eye chakra carry out its responsibility.

Moreover, keep in mind that your brow chakra is a heavenly instrument that once opened and intensified with reflection, can achieve experiences and understandings that will tenderly guide you and move you toward your most astounding development and advancement in life. The third eye is associated with duality which is a sort of discernment that restricts reality and is made exclusively by the psyche. When the third eye chakra is in amicability with the remainder of the chakras, it is said that an entryway towards otherworldly edification is opened. At the point when our third eye chakra is opened and well-balanced, we see existence with lucidity and have a stronger hold of our instincts. We also have a firm grasp on knowledge, mindfulness, and enthusiastic equalization. Then again, when our third eye chakra is blocked or imbalanced, we will in general battle with issues, such as closed-mindedness, skepticism, tension, discouragement, neurosis, and other dysfunctional behaviors or disposition issues.

Third eye chakra mending is the act of purging, opening, and adjusting the third eye chakra inside our bodies. Third eye chakra mending utilizes a wide scope of all-encompassing recuperating solutions for the body, brain, and soul. These cures incorporate practices, such as meditation, reflection, care, color treatment, sound treatment, yoga, self-healing, fragrance-based treatment, and others. The third eye chakra instructs us that death is nothing to fear - it is essential to grasp your time on this planet and after everything has been done, you will leave your body. Death is nevertheless a door leading to the next reality.

How To Successfully Open Your Third Eye

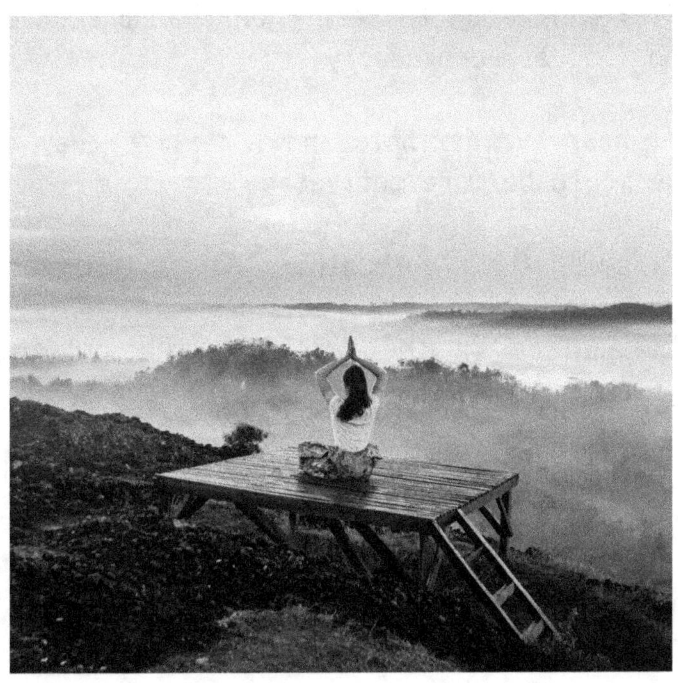

Confirmations or affirmations are phrases that target negative and constraining convictions and supplant them with increasingly positive convictions. They can be utilized to assist you with so many of your goals, from weight reduction to discovering love. So, it makes sense that they can likewise be utilized to adjust chakras.

When structuring third eye assertions, you need to concentrate on otherworldliness, your gut impulses, and the internal feeling of direction. Here are a few examples you can use. Don't hesitate to alter them until they feel right for you:

- "I pursue the lead of my instincts."

- "I realize how to settle on the correct choices, and I do as such easily."

- "I hear my instincts and I realize they will allow me to be more motivated."

- "I am on the right path."

- "I confide in the direction that my third eye gives me."

- "I have boundless conceivable outcomes that are accessible to me."

- "I am an instinctive individual, and I comprehend what is right for me."

- "My third eye is open and I am prepared to see my motivation."

In Hinduism, the third eye symbolizes a higher condition of cognizance through which you can see the world for what it truly is. Utilizing conventional reflection systems, you can open up this chakra and progressively illuminate comprehension of the universe around you. However, these aren't the only things that will allow you to open up your third eye chakra. In the earlier paragraphs, we have provided you with a brief introduction to what this chakra point is all about. As you may know, chakras are the energy focuses on your body. Basically, these are wheels of vitality that run along your spine. There are seven chakras, and each is associated with an alternate piece of your physical, mental, and otherworldly prosperity. Your third eye chakra is the 6th chakra. This is situated at the edge of your cerebrum, between your two eyes. It is directly over the extension of your nose. When you ruminate, attempt to concentrate your psyche on this chakra. It is in charge of helping you see the world for what it truly is.

o Choose a place for meditation

As you may already know, meditation is one of the best devices for achieving mindfulness. Earlier, we discussed what the third eye chakra is all about. By carrying more attention to your considerations, you will most likely have better access to the psychological lucidity that is related to the third eye. The central objective of reflection is to expedite the psyche to rest on one idea or item. It is critical to pick the appropriate surroundings where you feel great when you are starting to ponder or meditate. While a few people feel progressively serene and receptive when they are out in nature, this does not mean that it could work for you as well. On the off chance that this seems like you, you should seriously mull over contemplating outside. Discover a space that is the correct temperature and where you can sit without being aggravated by others. Indoor reflection is perfectly fine as well. Numerous individuals have an assigned reflection space in their home. This, for the most part, incorporates a pad or yoga mat that makes it increasingly agreeable to sit on the floor, and maybe a few candles and meditative music. Keep in mind that contemplation is an individual procedure. You ought to pick the surroundings that are for you.

o Pick a stance and focus on it

The next step would be to focus on your stance. The mind-body association is significant in meditation. The more physically agreeable you are, the simpler it will be to concentrate on your own contemplative thought. The best reflection stance is sitting leg over leg on the ground. In the event that you are accustomed to sitting on a chair, take some time every day to become acclimated to sitting on the floor. Over time, it will feel increasingly familiar. Moreover, other people use a pad or yoga mat to make sitting on the ground agreeable. Don't hesitate to utilize a few pads in the event that you discover this works better for you. Nevertheless, the closer you are to the ground, the better. On the off chance that you cannot simply bring yourself to sit on the floor due to certain body aches or whatnot, don' t stress about it. You can try what is known as the Walking Reflection. For certain individuals, the cadenced hints of their footsteps can be helpful in their meditative practice. When you' re doing this, be sure to walk slowly and gradually. Go about your way in a sense that you do not have any specific goal in mind as to where you are going.

o Choose a contemplation object

Then, you would want to pick a contemplation object. The purpose of picking one is to make it simpler to center the wandering mind. This will shield your considerations from any meanderings of the mind and will make your contemplation progressively powerful. Candles are a mainstream contemplation object. The flashing fire is anything but difficult to take a gander at and can console numerous individuals. Your contemplation object does not need to be close-by physically. Don't hesitate to picture a place like a sea or a lovely tree that you once observed when you were once driving by the countryside. Simply ensure you can obviously observe the item in your inner being.

o Choose a mantra

A mantra is a word or expression that you will continue to repeat during your meditative practice. You may state the mantra internally or out loud for anyone to hear. Your mantra ought to be something that is close to heart and important to you. Your mantra ought to be something that you need to incorporate into your psyche. For instance, you may rehash, "I choose to be happy." This will help fortify the possibility that you are going to concentrate on the inclination of being happy for the duration of the day. Another tip for when you're choosing a mantra is to pick only a single word. For instance, you could repeat the word "harmony." Nevertheless, whatever mantra you choose for your meditative practices, always make it a daily practice. Reflection is a kind of training. Figuring out how to effectively reflect by yourself is a procedure and it will require some time.

Moreover, it is best to ensure to go about it slowly. Start by contemplating for about two minutes, then move to meditate for about five minutes, and so forth. Before long, you will feel progressively good with the procedure and have the option to dedicate more opportunity to reflection every day. For beginners, it may be difficult to comprehend or even notice how your third eye is slowly opening itself. You will need to decipher your extrasensory observations with much lucidity as could reasonably be expected. Since we need enough vitality going through our entire body and enthusiastic framework to help a sound opening of unobtrusive channels of observation. At the point when the third eye gets actuated, the data that comes through might show up rather surprising, new, or just exasperating to the basic personality. It can enable us to open up unhindered thoughts and keep away from the normal negative manifestations of third enlightening; for example, the feeling of being perplexed or befuddled.

Situated between the temples and simply over the eye level, the third eye is related to instinct and knowledge as we have explained time and time again. In the human body, this chakra point is generally connected with the pituitary organ, just like that of the pineal organ. Organs and chakras are personally related as they speak to various degrees of substantial capacities; with the first being centered around the physical, the other on the unobtrusive enthusiastic level. The pituitary organ is viewed as the "master organ" in the human body since it controls the greater part of the various organs and their hormone generation. Shouldn't something be said about the pineal organ? Well, the pineal organ is situated in the mind, at a similar level as our eyes. Its association with the Ajna in Hinduism has for quite some time been researched by yogic conventions and present-day mysticism alike. They see this organ as a conceivable seat of the spirit and its improvement, a hotspot for supernatural encounters, as well as extrasensory recognition or clairvoyant capacities. This organ is generally viewed as responsible for creating melatonin and controlling our rest cycle, as well as our sexual development.

Moreover, to support your pineal organ and the enlivening of your third eye, the following points are things you can do:

Go outside and be one with nature. This is a good place to start because you want to allow your body to receive natural light. The next steps would include eating a proper and healthy diet consisting of the right kind of food for the pineal organ and those that can counter its calcification; for example, iodine, chlorella, apple juice, tamarind, and other natural products as it helps expel the excess amount of fluoride associated with the diminished pineal movement. Ponder; contemplation adjusts the movement of the sensory system and invigorates portions of the cerebrum that help the pineal organ. Spend time in the dark as it animates a sound action in the organ, as well as the generation of any related hormones. There are also explicit practices to initiate the third eye chakra, such as careful breathing that can quiet the brain and paved the way to the opening of your third eye. Nevertheless, being aware of your breathing takes into account purifying, yet additionally balances the chakra framework. The third eye is critical in imagining and dream review. Draw in and initiate your third eye chakra by maintaining a fantasy diary. It could be helpful to figure out how to enact and keep up your alpha and theta brainwaves. These cultivate frontal projection movement and set up your third eye and mind to be increasingly responsive.

Lastly, you can also acquaint basic oils with your home, shower, and body. Inconspicuous aromas can do some amazing things for opening, purging, and adjusting the body's chakras. To help recuperate and actuate your 6th chakra, think about attempting one or a blend of these fundamental oils: Roman or German chamomile, sandalwood, grapefruit, myrrh, and nutmeg.

Chapter 3:
Basics of Chakra Healing

What You Need To Know About Chakra Healing

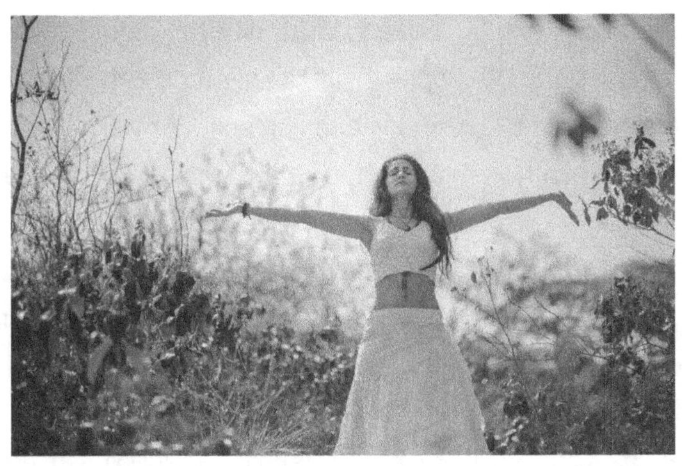

Chakra healing is an enormous part of the process of clearing up any chakra blockages in your body. Do remember that a chakra blockage or lopsidedness in one or a few of the seven main chakras can start mental, physical, or potentially spiritual infirmities. Despite whether you use chakra stones, gems, or another type of vibrational healing approach to reestablish chakra balance, being knowledgeable about chakra frameworks, their capacity, and the regions they administer can be useful. Moreover, balancing the chakras and healing the chakra framework requires you to be knowledgeable about the chakras and their capacities. While a fundamental chakra diagram outlines the essential seven chakras, did you know there are extra chakras to consider? As explained in the earlier paragraphs, there are over 114 chakra points in our body.

In fact, the more advanced students would start by discussing the 12 chakras and immediately meditating on them. Now, do keep in mind that there is more to meditation than merely repeating a mantra while you keep your eyes closed. There are also certain challenges faced by an individual when it comes to getting the hang of things in relation to meditative practice. For example, some would say that they are either too busy or too stressed to actually take the time from their schedule to fit in at least a five-minute meditation session. This can absolutely be valid if, for example, you have a long list of tasks to accomplish, such as having small kids and a nine-to-five work. Be that as it may, we are just discussing possibly around ten minutes per day - sometimes, even less. Majority of us invests more energy than the simple act of perusing the paper or surfing the web. It just seems as if we don't have the opportunity to meditate because, for the most part, we fill each minute with so many movements and never take the moment to catch our breath. There is no therapeutic solution for stress but meditation and reflection can probably come close. Nevertheless, the point that we are trying to make is that you need to warm up to the idea of meditation. Meditative practice is a sidekick to have all throughout your life, similar to an old companion you go to when you need motivation.

Moreover, there are also those who say, "I can't unwind, I just can't! Deadlines are making me insane!" Does this sound familiar? Well, these people are those that actually believe meditation to be pointless and simply a waste of time. The sad part is that they feel like they should prioritize their work - a great example of a source of stress - rather than spend the time to take a step back and meditate. The psyche is said to resemble a plastered monkey chomped by a scorpion, in light of the fact that similarly as a monkey jumps from branch to branch, so does the mind jumps starting with one thought then onto the next, always occupied and busy. When you come to sit still and attempt to calm your brain, you discover this hyper movement going on and it appears to be madly boisterous. It's quite new that you get to be mindful of it, much like the fear of the monkey being chomped by a scorpion. This experience of how the mind is so occupied is actually common and very typical. Long stretches of occupied personality, of making and looking after tasks and deadlines, of stress and the feeling of overwhelming anxiety; it's no wonder that the brain has no clue how to stay composed. It's not as though you can suddenly turn the brain off, yet the experience of stillness is collective. The more you sit still, the psyche ends up calmer. Each time you discover your brain is floating, wandering off into fantasy land, recollecting the past or preparing for the future, simply return to the now and return to this time. Sadly, gone are the days when we could vanish into a cavern and be left undisturbed until we feel the need to hunt for food or shelter again. Rather, mankind today needs to manage the sounds and burdens of our general surroundings.

A few people understand how advantageous meditative practice is even after only one session, yet the majority of us take longer — you may see a distinction following your first seven days of daily meditation; sometimes, this would last up to a month or so. This implies you need to believe that the procedure is enough to bring you what you want in life. You need to believe in its power even before you experience the benefits. Keep in mind that, in Japan, it can take 12 years to figure out how to perfect the art of origami. Being still occurs in a minute; however, it might take some time before that minute is truly up - henceforth, the requirement for this practice is one's patience and persistence. Additionally, it's difficult to come up short when you are meditating. There is no correct way to do it, and there's no wrong way to do it too. It's all up to you and what makes you feel alright. So, all you need to do is discover the way that works for you and keep at it. You can sit on the floor, sit in a chair, lie down, or walk around as you reflect; for example, you can do yoga or you can go about for a stroll as you contemplate the beauty of nature. You can also watch and assess the way you breathe; you can rehash a mantra; you can attempt to create a cherishing sense of thoughtfulness. Truly, there's so much you can do that meditative practice doesn't come in a one-size-fits-all step-by-step manual. In fact, this book is just a guide wherein you get to learn the basics of chakra meditation, but you are also given the freedom to alter most of the data presented here.

With this in mind, let's start to comprehend the process steps that will allow an individual to achieve clarity and a well-balanced chakra framework by discussing the process of energy healing.

What Is Energy Healing?

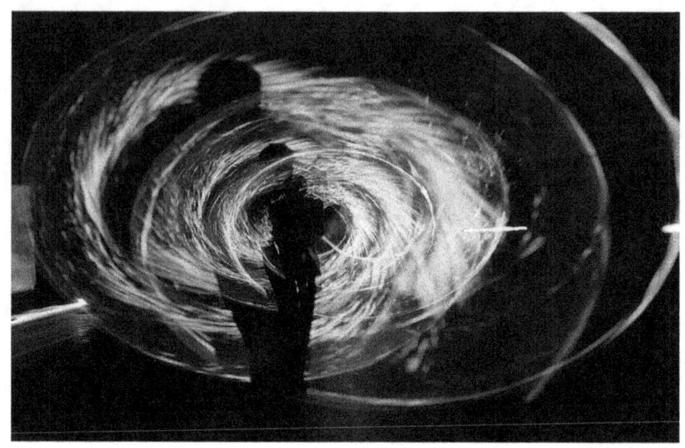

Energy healing was known and polished by practically all of the ancient societies and is presently being recently rediscovered by the West. Biomedical research is currently moving toward another model for the human body, which is known as the Energy Field Model. This is a similar model that Ancient China and Ancient India have based their way of thinking and their restorative frameworks upon; this includes the Ayurvedic and Yogic frameworks, the Acupuncture meridians, and so forth. This new model stems from the idea that life originated from electrical charges of energy. This thought brought about the concept that electromagnetic energy flows throughout the body. Moreover, scientists have also claimed that this particular energy pursues an organized way along the meridians. We've mentioned this earlier in the book but did not delve into much of the concept of Chi or Prana. Today, we have evidence of the presence of electrical fields, such as the EKG, EEG, and so on. Notwithstanding the dissemination of this energy, there is a power field of vitality in and around a human body, much like that of the magnetic field around a magnet. This field can be affected emphatically or adversely and it may very well be seen by certain well-gifted people. This so-called field is called "aura," which are human energy fields that emit colors that represent the inner flow of Chi. Thus, you may have heard of the saying, "Don't attack my space," whenever someone stands excessively close to you.

At this point, we have managed to discuss the basic concepts of the chakra system. Chakras are spinning vortexes of energy, arranged along the spinal segment. These are not physical but rather spiritual in nature. Another fundamental idea pertaining to the Energy Field Model is that - this vitality is certainly not a thoughtless or, as we state in prescription, supratentorial type of energy. Experts would like to look at this as a concentration of matter where it realizes what's going on and will endeavor to address it. If you're having a bad day because you had a failing grade on one of your tests, it will try to assess the situation and still bring out the best in you. If you are feeling under the weather, it will do its best to bring about self-recuperation. Of course, all of these is possible with the idea that your chakra points are balanced.

In Ayurvedic healing, there is the concept of the three doshas - Pitta, Vata, and Kapha. These are thought to lie at the center of this energy points or at the mind-body intersection. The brain is viewed as the center of all of this. This is the reason why the brain can impact an amazing effect on the distinct individual's wellbeing. This progression of vitality can be affected adversely, or even hindered, from multiple points of view. Poisons like pesticides, plastics, synthetic substances can obstruct its stream. Moreover, so can negative feelings. On another note, the techniques for treatment at the vibrational level are additionally too various to even think about mentioning them at all. Homeopathy, Ayurvedic and Chinese herbs, and sound, light, and color treatment, as well as meditation and yoga, are just some of the top things to do to achieve a well-balanced chakra framework.

So, what is Energy Healing exactly? All things considered, for the vast majority the idea of the concept of chakra, we are starting to rediscover through Quantum Physics that all issue - seen and concealed - is comprised of energy streams. This incorporates our physical bodies which are three dimensional, yet in addition and all the more significantly, the undetectable segments of ourselves which are alluded to by different names including an individual's spirit or soul. In this manner and in its most straightforward structure, Energy Healing is a technique for tuning in to one's inner self and the recuperation of the individual on a more spiritual level. To make things more clear, remember when we explained how meditation should address both the mind and the body? Well, for lack of a better term, chakra meditation highly focuses on the inner self, which comprises of the soul. Do note that with the healing of this inner self, the physical self is also healed because we have what we call the mind-body association. However, we are focusing on what chakra meditation can do as a part of one's journey to achieve a holistic healthy mind and body. Over time, you have learned that each of the chakra points has corresponding relationships with certain body parts. As a result, this may explain as to why some experts would rather opt to heal their inner self first, before diving into the use of other kinds of medication, which most likely only heals the physical self.

Truth be told, the idea of an all-inescapable power or vitality is an antiquated one, extending from China and Japan where it is known as Chi and Ki individually, to India where it is called Prana, to the Polynesian Islands where it is known as Mana. Additionally, in Nigerian spiritual practice, the term "Hurt" might be connected to an individual's general profound power or vitality. As the learning as to how our bodies have these energy fields had existed since the beginning of time, so too have strategies or frameworks of healing them which influence us on a vigorous level been created and used by ancient civilizations. For example, in the Hawaiian Islands, we have "Huna." In China, there is the practice of Acupuncture and Acupressure as a means to target specific chakra points. In India, there are different structures like the process of "Pranic Healing." Japan has what they call "Reiki," which is a non-intrusive and delicate treatment which we will investigate further in the succeeding books.

The truth is that, whether or not you believe in the existence of these chakra points, you are actually acknowledging that there is a field or force within you via the way you react to certain scenarios. The trick here is to notice the signs that would back up these concepts. Most of the time, people seem to merely neglect these signs. As a result, they tend to blame other things for why they are acting this way or why certain things are happening to them. Well, if at this point, you are still skeptic, read the following statements to achieve more clarity regarding this topic.

1. You've just met someone and, for reasons you can't generally clarify, you either extremely like this person or you hate them. You have never met this person before and he/she has not done anything to you to merit your blessing or your objection towards their existence.

2. You stub your toe or hit your head, and your immediate reaction was to put your hand where it hurts.

3. You become distinctly and incredibly mindful that something isn't right with a friend or a family member, yet you are not with them or you have not contacted them recently.

These three models are simply basic events which we may underestimate and give no additionally thought, despite the fact that there is no conspicuous method to clarify what is occurring - but there's an explanation to all of these and figuring out the answer would depend on how well you are acquainted with your body's chakra system.

The Power And Benefits Of Energy Healing

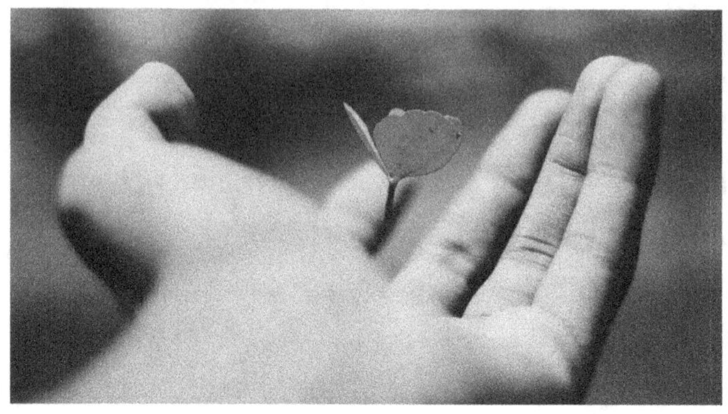

Reiki, which is a type of energy healing process, is also considered as a type of elective treatment generally alluded to as vitality mending. It developed in Japan in the late 1800s and is said to include the exchange of general vitality from the professional's palms to their patient. So, as compared to what we have been telling you, the healing and balancing of one's chakra system can be done with an expert. In vitality recuperation, it is important to recognize how this practice has been utilized for quite a long time in different structures. Promoters state it works with the vitality fields around the body. However, there has been some debate that encompasses Reiki, in light of the fact that it is difficult to demonstrate its adequacy through logical methods. Be that as it may, numerous individuals who get Reiki state it works and its notoriety is definitely expanding. In fact, a 2007 overview demonstrates that, in the United States of America, about 1.2 million adults have attempted Reiki. More than 60 emergency clinics have even confirmed to offer Reiki administrations to their patients. As for its terminologies, the word "Reiki" signifies "universal energy." It originates from the Japanese words "rei," which means "general," and "ki," which means life energy. Thus, if you want to further understand what energy healing or chakra recuperation is all about, you may have better luck at understanding Reiki. Luckily, we will devote an entire segment to Reiki healing in the books the succeeds this one. For this book, we will focus on the more basic concepts. Besides, much like the fact that you need to start with your root chakra as a basis, you also need to start with the basic principles of chakra meditation.

As indicated by experts, vitality can stagnate in the body where there has been physical damage or perhaps torment. In time, these energy points will lead to a more serious ailment. Those who are considered to be expert at chakra healing may recommend various ways like needle therapy or pressure point massage. Improving the progression of vitality around the body, as explained by these professionals, can empower one's self, diminish one's suffering and torment, speed up self-recuperation, and decrease the various symptoms of sickness. Again, we could not stress this enough that it is important to find the right method for you to achieve a well-balanced chakra system. Moreover, since Reiki healing is somehow similar to the majority of the chakra healing processes, let's start to use it as a basis for our comparison.

Reiki has been around for many years. Its present structure was first created in 1922 by a Japanese Buddhist called Mikao Usui, who allegedly showed 2,000 individuals the Reiki technique at the time when he was alive. The training spread to the United States of America through Hawaii during the 1940s, and afterward to Europe during the 1980s. It normally alludes to hands-on-body healing. It is best done in a tranquil setting; however, there is a possibility to perform it anywhere as long as the practitioner is well-equipped. Basically, what you need to learn about this process is that the existence of Chi in our body allows the practitioner to heal the other person from various illnesses, discharge blockages, poisons, and even ease their torment. Furthermore, it can also assist you in making better decisions in your life, become progressively mindful, and be able to be more in tune with your body. As a result, you will pay more attention to your body's needs. On a psychological level, this process can assist you with witnessing your contemplations and negative thoughts. When you become mindful of your musings, you have the ability to transform them. This isn't about positive reasoning. In fact, this is more tied in with finding out about your musings and getting to be mindful of your contemplations, so you can deliberately settle on a choice whether the considerations are serving you well or not. On an otherworldly level, it can assist you with loving and acknowledging yourself and have self-empathy and sympathy for other people.

The Relationship Between Chakras And Your Health

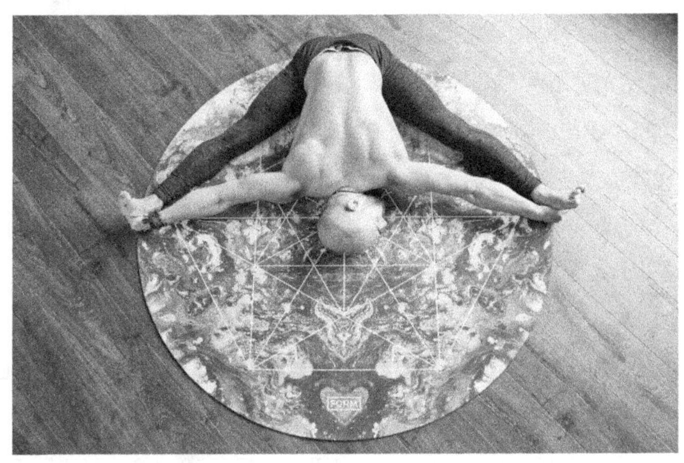

Sickness is reproduced in the body not just because of hereditary change or poor karma in one' s wellbeing. It is also not exclusively gained from smoking or eating an unhealthy diet. In fact, most would believe that for an infection to occur, it must be associated with corruption in the brain, which directly affects the condition of your body. The way one feels rationally or one's frame of mind can definitely have an impact on the wellbeing of the body.

At this point, we have already established that there are energy points in our body from the bottom of your back to the top of your head. This entire system is considered as the chakra framework. There is a process to be followed if one wants to achieve holistic health, which pertains to both mental and physical health of a person. Moreover, we have also tackled as to how different types of chakra recuperation, such as Reiki and Acupuncture, believes in the idea the Chi runs through our body. The manipulation of this Chi can affect how we think and how we see the world; thus, it can also affect how our bodies function. With all of these in mind, anyone who wishes to achieve holistic health must also be knowledgeable of the different chakra points - well, at least the seven main ones. Understand that one's point of view, the words that one uses in ordinary discussions and the individual contemplations and emotions that are kept in the darkest corners of the mind assume a job in the trustworthiness of the bodies health.

As you may know, these chakra points each portray an exact degree of cognizance inside the person's body and would often control our mental state just as our association with the physical and profound world, as well as the energies from above. Chi enters the crown chakra from the universe, from that point it descends each chakra bringing new vitality and recuperating by refining negative feelings and expelling negative vitality related with them. At the root chakra, the vitality returns and climbs up the body being discharged at the crown and reappearing to the universe again. Even though Chi enters from the crown chakra, we could not stress this enough that you must start your meditative practices from bottom to top so as to achieve a kind of grounding. Nevertheless, you can only imagine how a single blocked chakra point won' t allow the Chi to pass through. Their equalization is an impression of the parity of the body. Like a biological system that requirements to work synergistically at each level so as to keep up consonant parity, so does the need for each chakra to be open and well-balanced.

With this in mind, let's take a look as to how each chakra point affects or contributes to our holistic health. What are the illnesses or body parts that each chakra is associated to? You'll find the answers to this question in the succeeding points. Before you start with any meditative practice, it is actually highly recommended to learn about each of these chakras because most of your meditation will center on how you can picture a particular chakra opening. If you don't know anything about the chakras, then you wouldn't be able to achieve a clear mental image of what you want to open.

- **The Root Chakra**

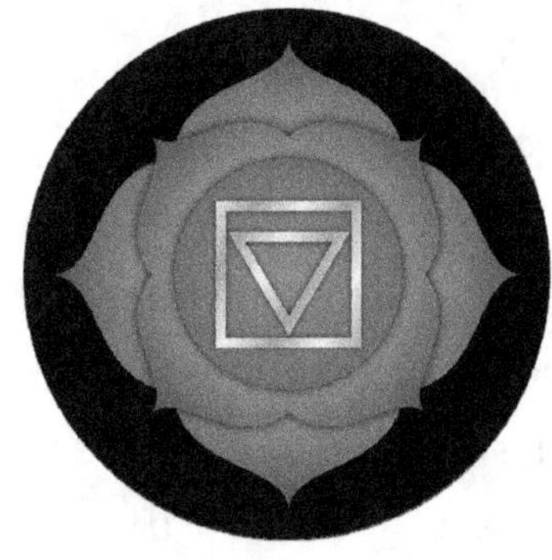

The first chakra is usually alluded to as the root chakra and is situated at the perineum. It is calculated south from an individual's body, which symbolizes the entrance toward the earth. A little recap of what we have discussed in the earlier chapters, the first chakra impacts the rectal and genital regions, the coccyx, the male organ, and even the bladder. Vitality to the legs, knees, and feet may likewise be affected by the first chakra.

- **The Sacral Chakra**

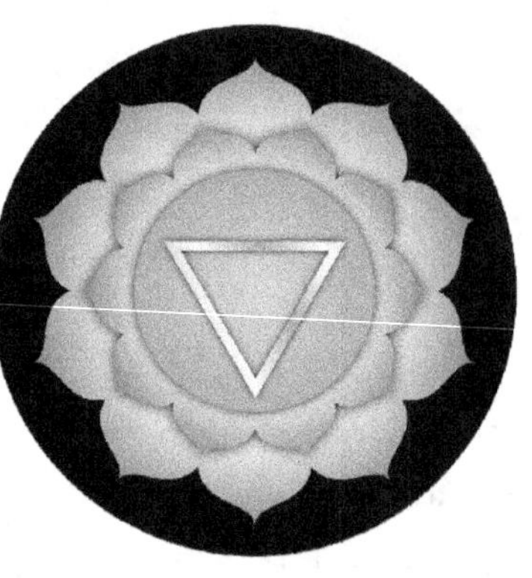

The second chakra impacts the female regenerative organs, the internal organ and colon, the bones and muscles of the pelvic zone, and the sacral zone. The second chakra impacts one's ability to connect and converse with someone else, a particular circumstance, or experience on a passionate and enthusiastic level. This influences ones capacity to be physically or vigorously open to sensation. The second chakra also impacts sexual fascination, enthusiastic holding, and sexual association.

- **The Solar Plexus Chakra**

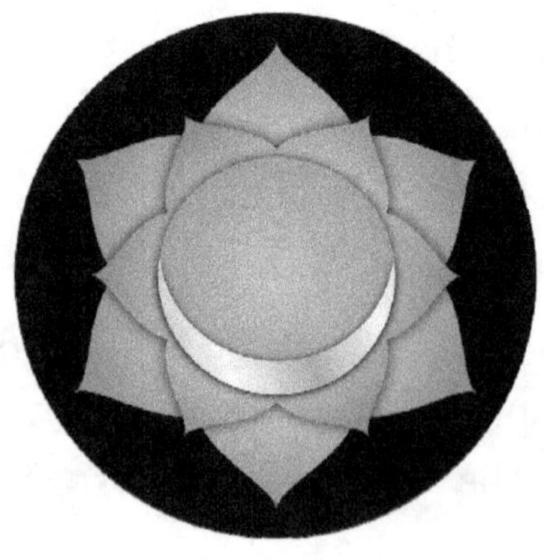

The third chakra is regularly alluded to as the solar plexus chakra and is situated beneath the breastbone. This chakra impacts the nerve bladder, liver, spleen, stomach, small digestive system, kidneys, pancreas, and the lower back. The third chakra impacts self-acknowledgment and affirmation, association with oneself, and such. This includes the capacity to perceive and bolster one's needs, qualities, feelings and wants, just as one's capacity to speak their mind. It impacts one's capacity to discover satisfaction and happiness throughout everyday life, and one's feeling of pride and self-esteem.

- **The Heart Chakra**

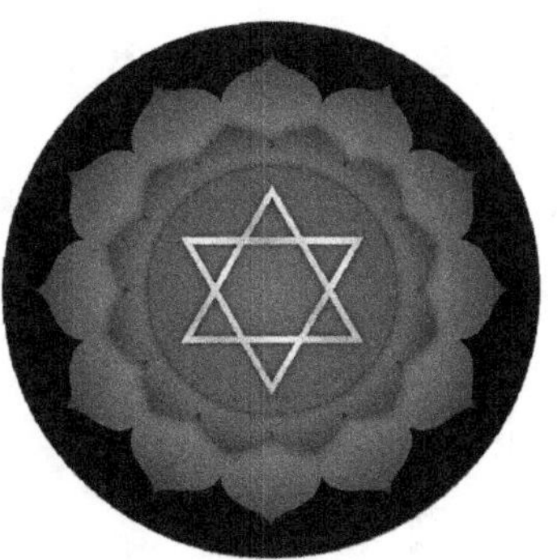

The fourth chakra is usually referred to as the heart chakra. As the name suggests, this chakra impacts the heart, mid-thoracic vertebrae, lungs, arms, and bosoms. This chakra impacts one's capacity to cherish certain moments and relationships, as well as connect with other people. The fourth chakra is the combination of all your life experiences, where an individual coordinates understanding and transmute this experience into information, knowledge, harmony, pardoning, and discharge.

- ## The Throat Chakra

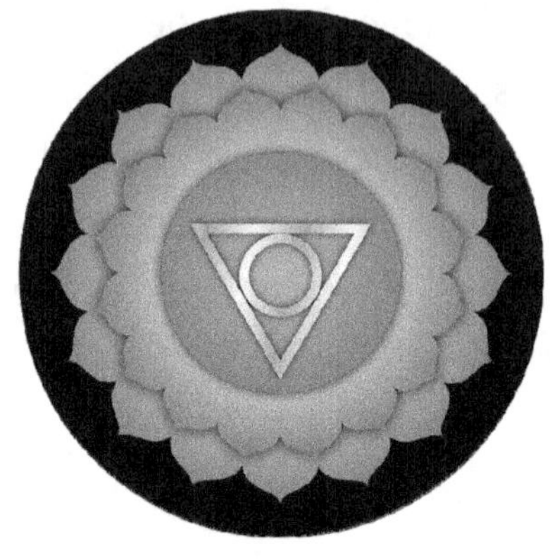

The fifth chakra is ordinarily alluded to as the throat chakra and is situated at the fourth cervical vertebrae, in the focal point of the throat. This is simply the focal point of inventiveness, articulation, and correspondence. It permits or disallows one to bring what is back to front, offering a voice to oneself and permitting imaginative energies, thoughts, and dreams to show. It impacts one's receptiveness to relationships and correspondence with others. The fifth chakra is an amazing focus, as it can permit or square the progression of vitality all through the vitality framework.

- ## The Third Eye Chakra

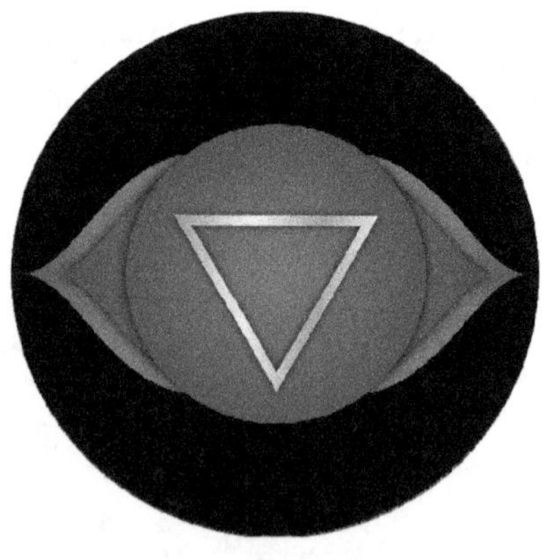

The sixth chakra is regularly known as the third eye chakra and is situated in the mid-temple. This is probably one of the more famous chakra points as it has been associated with various mystical powers. Physically, the sixth chakra impacts the eyes,

88

mind, pineal organ, and the sinuses. The sixth chakra impacts mental lucidity, otherworldly level knowing, and vision. It impacts the brain's capacity to know what is unmistakably there. The sixth chakra also impacts an individual's profound internal knowing and understanding that is often dependent on the familiarity of one's genuine self; just as one's capacity to see what is actually present in this reality and time.

- **The Crown Chakra**

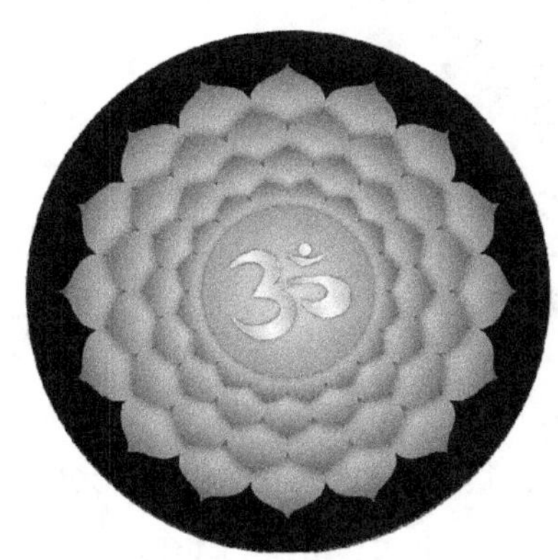

The seventh chakra is known as the crown chakra and is situated at the highest point of the head, which symbolizes our bodies' opening so that the universe is able to send us messages. The seventh chakra is an otherworldly focus and impacts one's transparency and association with the nonphysical components of the universe, keeping profound mindfulness in one's cognizance. It impacts one's association with the divine source, bringing the sentiment of being profoundly associated and bolstered all through one's everyday experience. It influences one's capacity to acknowledge their existence as an unbounded being, which brings a more noteworthy consciousness to one's self.

Top 25 Benefits Of Clearing And Balancing Your Chakras

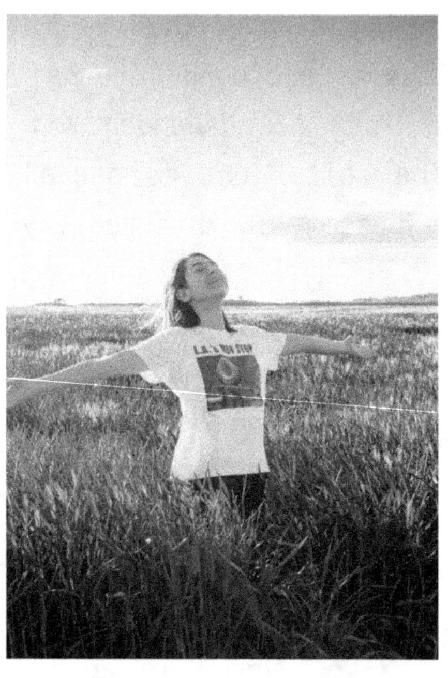

Chakra healing poses various advantages that can occur at any level. These can be emotional, yet are frequently inconspicuous. These can also happen promptly, yet frequently appear later, even after the healing session has been long finished. Nevertheless, when it comes to the true benefits of balancing all of your chakra points may seem ordinary, but put all of these together and you are guaranteed to achieve wellbeing that allows you to truly enjoy life for what it is - no stress, no anxiety, and no worries. With that in mind, here are the top benefits you can expect once you have cleared all of your blocked chakra points.

1.   A more prominent feeling of being healthy.
2.   A profound feeling of harmony and quiet.
3.   A faster capability to heal not only your physi-
     cal injuries, but also your emotional, spiritual,
     and mental worries.
4.   The arrival of profound, endless muscle pres-
     sure.
5.   Alleviation of uneasiness.
6.   Access to financial wisdom and stability.
7.   Improved sense and ability to open yourself up
     to what's been troubling you.
8.   Alleviation and improved protection from inter-
     minable gloom or loneliness.
9.   Improved innovativeness, imaginative creation,
     and critical thinking.
10. Improved sense of knowledge.
11. Improved individual development, as well as oth-
     erworldly advancement.
12. Intense detoxification of negative thoughts and
     feelings.
13. Improved mental clearness.
14. Improved patience.
15. Improved ability to control your tantrums and
     outbursts.
16. Clearing up of any blocked chakra point.
17. Improved ability to communicate and express your
     inner desires and thoughts.
18. Establishment of one's sense of identity
     through self-reflection.
19. Receipt of universal support or motivation to
     further fulfill one's goals and objectives in
     life.

20. Improved ability to manifest your goals and objectives in life without the need to belittle or dominate others.
21. Deeper and well-rested night's sleep.
22. Openness to spontaneity and pleasure.
23. Openness to positive feelings, such as grounding, security, and stability.
24. Removal of any remaining bad energy stored in the body.
25. A heightened sense of intuition.

If you are to notice the above-mentioned items, all of these are mostly interrelated, much like how the sixth chakra is connected to the other five chakras and vice versa, these benefits are only achieved if you are able to clear the blockages on all chakra points. Yes, it is impossible to experience a heightened sense of intuition when one or two chakra points are balanced, but to truly accept what the universe has to offer, you must open your crown chakra, which is the last point to open. Remember, when achieving holistic health and mindfulness, always start with the root chakra.

At the point when the physical body is under proceeded with pressure, the chakras won't work appropriately. The way to recuperating is to address the underlying driver of the confusion, not simply the side effects. It is essential to know that the indications may not show in the place of the reason.

Chapter 4:
Basic Self-Healing Techniques:
How To Work With Your Chakras

Getting To Know Your Chakras Through Visualization

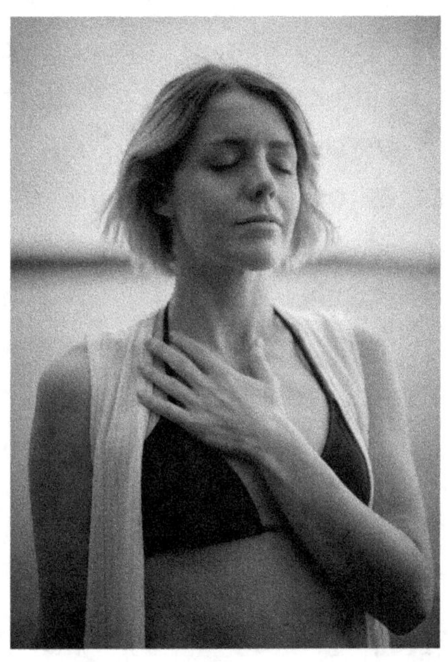

When it comes to chakra meditation, we would like to let you in on a well-known fact that most beginners fail to acknowledge - chakra meditation alone won't help you achieve a well-balanced chakra system. You need additional techniques and the help of various tools. While it is true that chakra meditation is fairly simple, it can also be a challenge, especially if you are not utilizing the right materials, but we're getting ahead of ourselves. Let's start with something basic - the proper way of visualizing the chakra centers. As you may have noticed in the previous chapters, we would often let you envision an intense light overpowering you from a particular part of your body; typically, the location of a specific chakra. This is a type of perception activity that can greatly help you unblock certain energy centers in the body. Most of the time, it is better to picture an image or scenery that calms you. Then, allow your mind to drift. There's no point in forcing certain images to come upon you. When it comes to meditation, forcing your mind to go blank is almost always a bad idea. Start by allowing your mind to drift. Even though there is a need to concentrate on the intense light that we've mentioned earlier, each time you catch your mind wandering, don't give yourself a mental slap in the face; simply bring yourself back to the image of the light. Sooner or later, you'll get the hang of things.

Begin by finding an area or space where you feel comfortable, enabling your body and psyche to unwind for quite a while. Welcome yourself to investigate whatever will enable you to be progressively present and in the moment. There are those that like to put on music or a guided recording of a meditation tutorial; whatever it is, as long as it brings you harmony and peace, you're good to go. Now, the next step would include you setting down serenely on your back. Tune into your breathing by setting your left hand on your heart and your correct hand on your stomach. You can bend your knees if you think it will help you lie down more comfortable. Then, start to take fuller and deeper breaths in and out through your nose. Again, focus on your breathing. Continue this practice for a couple more minutes and, when you're ready and when you've got the hang of things, start to envision a white light filling the space in your stomach and heart and, as you breathe out, imagine this white light transmitting all through your whole body from head to toe. When you complete the cycle, unwind for a couple of minutes and afterward complete the contemplation, by avowing you are solid, adjusted, and settled.

Congratulations! What you just did is an example of a very basic visualization exercise. It may sound easy enough, but you would know that you're getting good at it if you can quite your mind and intently focus on the white light for more than five minutes. Truly, visualization is a significant part of chakra meditation. It may very well be utilized as a type of self-reflection, as an imaginative method to show your fantasies and reveal your true desires, a way to manifest your objectives in life out into the universe, and an amazing asset for changing negative energy into a more positive one. Your intuitive personality is exceptionally responsive to visual pictures, and your creative mind can be utilized as an amazing asset to reconstruct your subliminal personality and mend any physical or mental subject matters that are influencing your life.

Inventive perception or guided representation is a ground-breaking and viable strategy you can use for opening, clearing, enacting, or even adjusting the vitality of each chakra point. Since each chakra speaks to an alternate part of your physical being, you can ponder the physical area and shade of each chakra by utilizing inventive representation for better outcomes. Our energy centers are basically turning vortices of light. This light is very much needed to sustain life. Ever since the beginning of time, our ancestors acknowledged the fact that such a system exists within our very selves.

Keeping up a solid and adjusted chakra framework is essential. Allow yourself the chance to assess what your physical body and spiritual mindset are passing on to you; better yet, what the universe is trying to tell you. Notwithstanding clearing and adjusting your chakras, it is significant and valuable to reinforce them through various techniques and tools beyond mere visualization, such as gemstones, colors, and the type of music you listen to. We should start by giving a concise outline of the chakra framework and how they work. You already know the location of the seven basic chakra centers. Chakra points are vitality vortexes that live in each and everyone' s bodies and tend to transfer the energy within us between the three entities that make up an individual. Our physical body, astral body, and mental body - these are the three entities that you should pay attention to. Charka focuses basically move vitality between these entities, by raising or dropping the recurrence of the vitality as required. Chakra points are in charge of your characteristics and, with a balanced chakra system, your physical and mental state are in parity too. So, since we already have a comprehension of chakra centers, how about we dive into the representation reflection system of this framework, which can be utilized to open and further balance these centers.

Each chakra point is related to a specific shading, and by utilizing this data alongside the intensity of fixation and perception, one can help animate a specific chakra and help it in clearing any blockages. The following is the shading diagram that rundowns the specific colors related to each chakra point. Every one of these hues should then be utilized, as depicted in the reflection content beneath it. Do note that the below-mentioned list can help you further your goals in achieving a well-balanced chakra system. Remember, these colors can be imbued in what you wear, what you eat, and the objects you associate with.

o The Root Chakra Color: Red

o The Sacral Chakra Color: Orange

o The Solar Plexus Chakra Color: Yellow

o The Heart Chakra Color: Green

o The Throat Chakra Color: Blue

o The Third Eye Chakra Color: Indigo

o The Crown Chakra Color: Violet

Now, let's proceed to combine the two concepts that were previously discussed - visualization and the use of chakra color correspondences. In the first part of this chapter, you were taught how to envision this white light that is slowly taking over you. Well, with the additional knowledge of the chakra colors, you can target a particular energy center by focusing on its corresponding color. For example, when achieving holistic health, you would want to start with the root chakra, which is energized by the color red. Since this chakra point is located at the bottom of your spine, envision - instead of white light - red light that is slowly emanating for where the root chakra should be.

This particular chakra meditative technique has its effect throughout the whole chakra framework; however, on the off chance that you are keen on opening and adjusting only one specific chakra, you can essentially concentrate on that particular energy center. This strategy for chakra adjusting is exceptionally viable, yet one should utilize it wisely, as one ought to be physically ready to deal with the expanded vitality stream that can happen when chakras are enacted and opened. Continue to take deeper breaths and try to picture other correspondences that would help get a much clearer image in your mind. If you're having a hard time doing this, the below details on each energy center may be useful for this practice.

- **The Root Chakra**

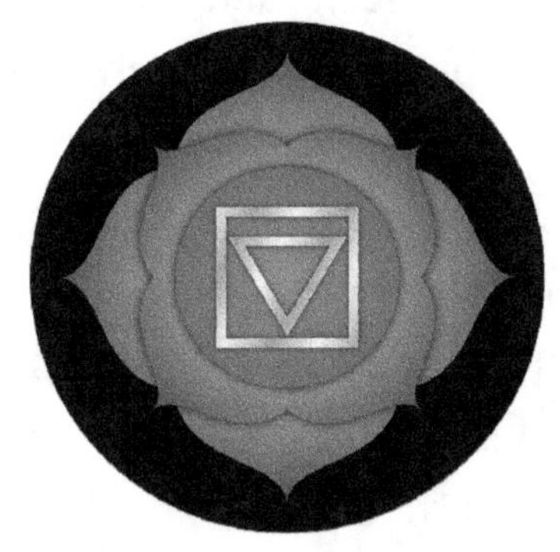

The root or base chakra is related to one's survival needs alongside the lower vibrational energies of stress, dread, question, lament, blame, and disgrace. It is our establishment and the association with the physical plane. To adjust and reinforce this chakra point, always make it a habit of incorporating the color red into your daily lives. This can be achieved through various ways. One example is by doing the following: wear red garments, eat red sustenance, such as raspberries, apples, strawberries, red pepper, tomatoes, and watermelon. On another note, you can also try to envision what you are eating or drinking as red and work with red precious stones; for example, garnet and jasper, or any of the establishing gems, including hematite.

- ## The Sacral Chakra

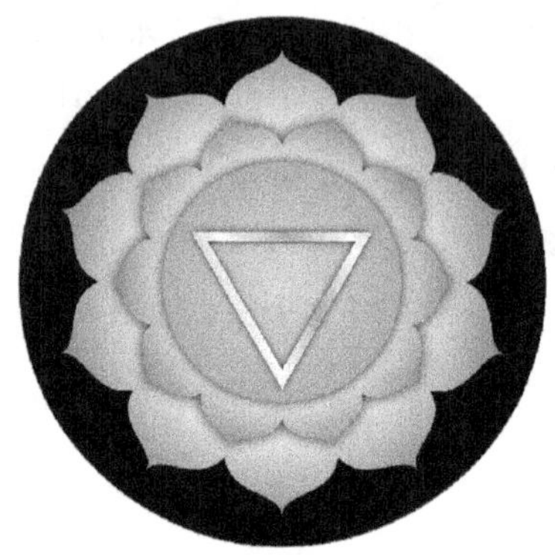

The sacral chakra often corresponds to the lively color of orange and is corresponded with imagination, motivation, and sexuality. Physical organs incorporated by this chakra point are as follows: the kidneys, lower intestine, liver, bladder, testicles, and ovaries. To adjust and reinforce this chakra point, it is important to work and utilize its corresponding color, which is orange. To achieve this and further bring about a balanced sacral chakra, try wearing orange apparel, consume orange sustenance, such as oranges, orange pepper, melons, apricots, carrots, sweet potatoes, and butternut squash, or envision what you are consuming - either eating or drinking - as something of orange color and work with orange precious stones; for example, carnelian, topaz, and orange calcite.

- ## The Solar Plexus Chakra

The solar plexus chakra often corresponds to the happy color of yellow. Physical organs incorporated by this chakra point are as follows: The stomach, liver, kidneys, and adrenal

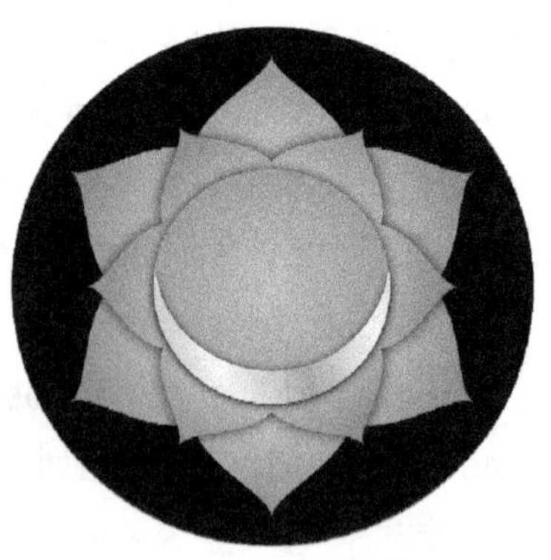

glands, which are identified with our will, individual power, and character. To adjust and fortify this energy center, work with the shading yellow and wear yellow attire. Make it a habit to eat squash, bananas, pears, pineapple, corn, or lemons. During your chakra meditation, you can use gemstones like the tiger's eye, yellow tourmaline, yellow calcite, or citrine.

- **The Heart Chakra**

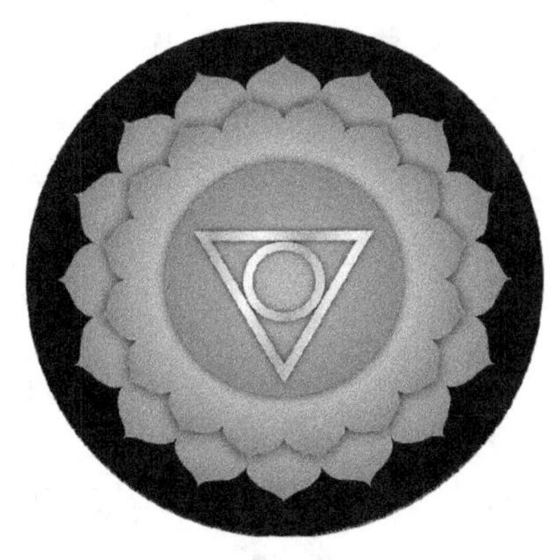

The heart chakra is associated with the color green. It is related with adoration and love for the self, as well as other people, and other similar feelings. To adjust and reinforce this energy point, work with the shading green and incorporate it into what you wear. Eat your green vegetables like cucumbers, broccoli, green beans, cabbage, green pepper, celery, lettuce, limes, kale, avocadoes, and peas. Also, it would greatly help you when meditating on your heart chakra to work with amazonite, aventurine, and chrysoprase.

- **The Throat Chakra**

The throat chakra is associated with the color blue and is considered as your voice - the territory of corre-

spondence and self-articulation. This chakra point is often associated with our respiratory system; thus, the or-
gans governed by the throat
chakra includes the thyroid organ, mouth, jaw, teeth, tongue,
and throat. To adjust and reinforce this energy point, wear
blue clothing and eat blue sus-

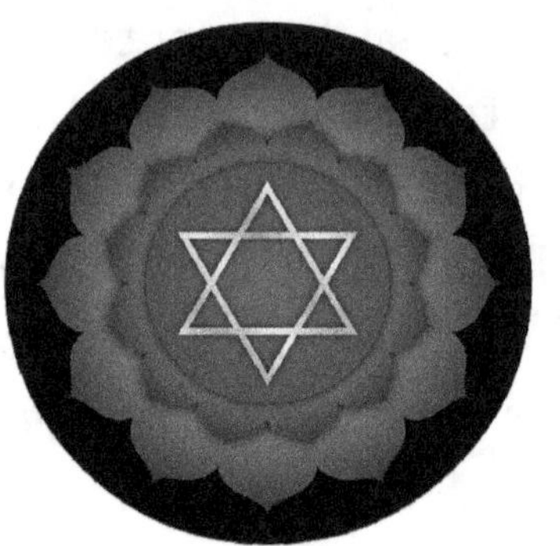

tenances, such as blueberries, or picture what you are
eating or drinking as something of the color blue. Some
of the gemstones you can use to represent the throat
chakra are as follows: sodalite, lapis lazuli, blue
lace agate, and blue calcite.

- **The Third Eye Chakra**

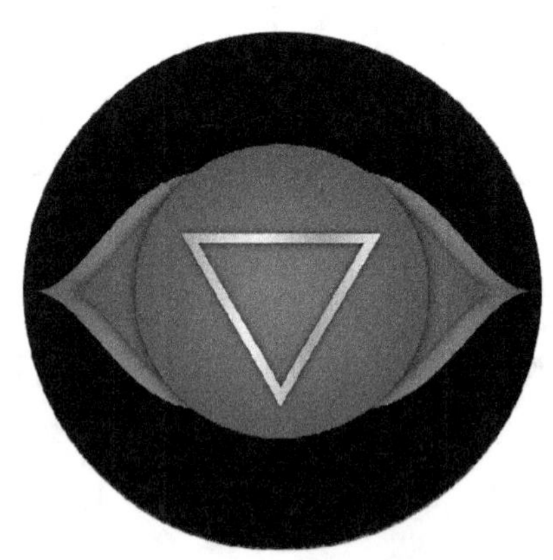

The third eye chakra is associated with the color violet
or indigo. Moreover, this is
your region of instinct and
profound mindfulness. The
physical body organs governed
by this chakra are the pituitary organ and pineal glands.
To adjust and reinforce this

energy point, wear purple garments or eat purple suste-
nances, such as eggplant, purple grapes, plums, and
purple cabbage. Moreover, when meditating, use amethyst
and purple fluorite.

- **The Crown Chakra**

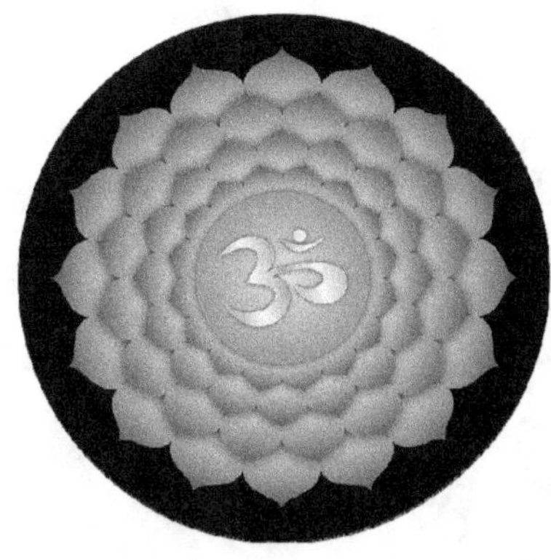

The crown chakra is associated with the color white and is your source of vitality from the universe. Much like the other chakras, to adjust and fortify this one, you must wear white attire and eat white nourishments, such as white onions, cauliflower, coconut, garlic, and mushrooms. Use amethyst crystals, gem quartz, and clear tourmaline and opal for when you are meditating.

How To Re-Align Your Entire Chakra System

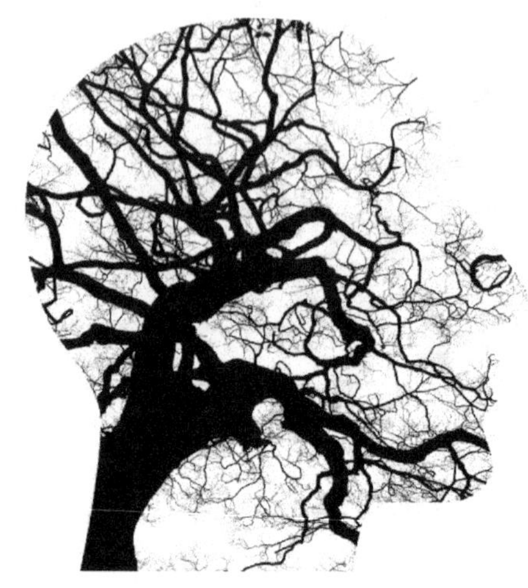

In case you're feeling down, lacking in vitality, discouraged, or overpowered by the feeling that you are
undesirable, it's probable that your chakras are unbalanced. Keeping up a sound body and mind that are in
synced with each other is a challenging task. Adjusting
your chakras brings about a well-established framework
with which you can restore your body and awareness back
to homeostasis, and keep it that way. Note that homeostasis is a state of equilibrium between the various
elements that are maintained by your physiological processes. Nevertheless, this part of the book will focus
on how you can align your entire chakra system. Over
the past chapters, we have been focusing on your individual energy centers. We may have mentioned how it is
important to start with the root chakra and move your
way up toward the crown chakra when attempting to establish a holistic state of mind and body, but this

isn't even the beginning of it. There are certain steps that you need to be aware of and follow so that you will end up with an aligned chakra system.

Since the chakras in your body are responsible for giving you energy and power that will help you go about your day-to-day activities, they can ostensibly play a persuasive job in directing your feelings and psychological well-being. In case you're experiencing any of the accompanying issues, it could be because of an issue with one or two of your chakras. Together, your chakras speak to your whole self - on a physical, mental, and even spiritual level. Thus, they give the methods and capability by which you can use to accomplish or achieve things in your life. By dedicating only a couple of minutes to effectively envision and support each of your chakras, you can improve every aspect of yourself. This time will be dedicated to a couple of minutes of concentrating your mindfulness on every one of the seven chakras. You will, without a doubt, advance the traits it speaks to. Odds are, in the event that you haven't been living under a rock for the past decade, you've known about yoga. Yoga, as it occurs, draws quite a bit of its mantra from the chakra framework. Truth be told, numerous cutting edge types of contemplation infer quite a bit of their substance from this comprehension of vitality stream between the major chakras. These frameworks would recognize that your awareness is spread over each of the seven chakras and that adjusting them all brings a condition of amicability and prosperity. In this sense, adjusting your chakras resembles being in a condition of contemplation, constantly enabling you to accomplish a good life.

There are a lot of manners by which you can approach the process of chakra alignment as a whole — this strategy is deeply rooted in the techniques of ancient civilizations. Since you have been equipped with the basics of what each of the seven chakras corresponds to, it is now time to bring them all together. You've learned how to meditate earlier - deep breaths while lying down with your hands on your heart and stomach - and you've also familiarized yourself with how the white light can be changed into a specific color in which a particular chakra point can represent. What you need to do now is to visualize the first chakra, the one at the base of your spine, and utilizing your creative mind by picturing all of the associations to that of the root chakra - color, organs, foods, color of your clothing, and more. Envision broadening this chakra to the width of your body. Even though the root chakra is often associated with the part at the bottom of the spine, we would want you to picture the light expanding until it is able to take over your entire body. However, you must this vortex precisely at the inside line of your body and at the base of the spine. Then, you proceed to envision the second chakra. Be sure to repeat the same process steps as you did with the root chakra. Next, the third chakra. Notice what feels distinctive as you are adjusting these vitality points. Proceed with the fourth, fifth, sixth, and seventh chakra. Take a couple of minutes to just lie there and absorb the sentiment of being whole. Try doing this consistently and you'll sure to get the hang of it. Soon, you'll be able to do it without forcing too much on picturing the light.

Common Symptoms Of Unbalanced Chakras

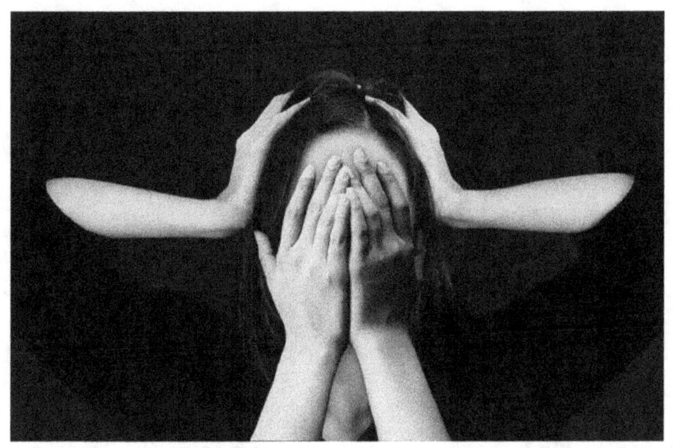

Have you been feeling down lately? Is it accurate to say that you are committing senseless errors at work? Is it accurate to say that you are wiped out for the third week straight? Albeit any number of things could be the clarification for these upsetting conditions, they could likewise be characteristic of unevenness in your chakra framework. Now that we've established what chakras are, the importance of the upkeep of your chakra system, the seven main chakras, their correspondences in terms of color, gemstones, music, and such, and the proper way of visualization when it comes to chakra meditation, let us now proceed to figure out which of the chakras are unbalanced. Moreover, it's now time to start asking the more specific set of questions? Is there a need to balance only one energy center? Can I balance both at the same time? What happens if I attempt to balance the crown chakra before the root chakra? What are some of the common symptoms of an unbalanced chakra?

Let's take it one at a time, shall we? Yes, your chakra system should be well-balanced so that you are able to receive the universe's energy, the same energy that will allow you to live a holistic life - both mind and body. On the other hand, you can balance only one chakra or the entire system, as long as you do it one by one, which leads us to the next question: What happens if I attempt to balance the crown chakra before the root chakra? Well, if you do so, you wouldn't have proper grounding as the root chakra is considered as the energy point that provides us with the ability to become much more stable in life and in the things we do. There is a high chance that you will not succeed at opening up the other six chakras if you were not able to achieve a well-balanced root chakra. Of course, there are those who - even before starting with their entire chakra journey - already have a balanced chakra point or two. If this is the case, then you can proceed on to the next chakra point that you wish to open or take care of. The tricky part here is knowing which of the seven main chakra points need to be balanced? Thus, we arrive at the common symptoms of an unbalanced chakra.

- **The Root Chakra**

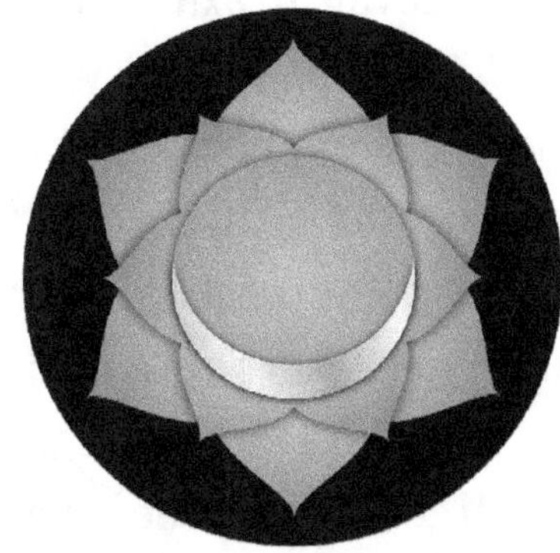

This chakra, which is physically situated at the feet, legs, and "roots" of your being, is associated with the element earth. You would know that your root chakra is unbalanced if you may experience pain and stiffness in your feet and legs. You may also experience aches in your hamstrings.

- **The Sacral Chakra**

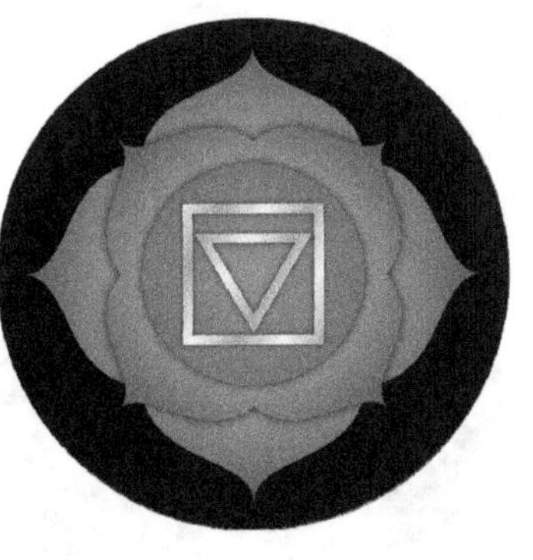

On the off chance that you are encountering any of the accompanying indications, you may have an unbalanced sacral chakra: pain and stiffness in your low back and hips. Moreover, if you notice your loss of creative mind or lack of innovativeness, out of touch with feelings and emotions toward others, and sexual and regenerative issues, then you may want to focus your meditation on the sacral chakra.

- ## The Solar Plexus Chakra

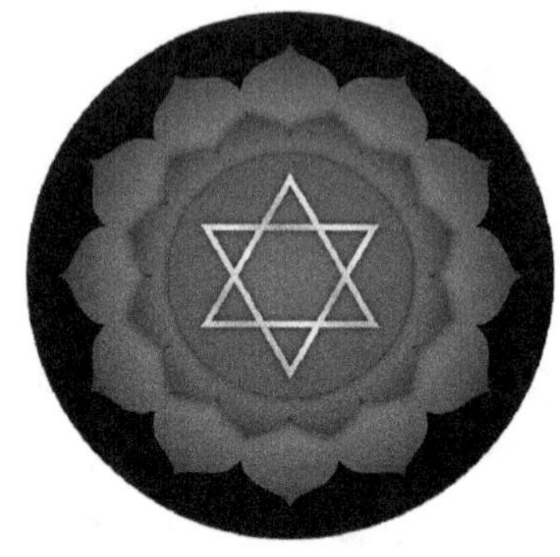

This solar plexus chakra, which is physically situated at the guts, is associated with the element fire. The solar plexus chakra is related to the majority of your contemplations and sentiments about yourself. This chakra is about your relationship with yourself. In the event that you are encountering any of the accompanying indications, you may have an irregularity in the solar plexus chakra: digestive issues and stomach aches, low confidence, overinflated self-esteem, and inability to finish objectives or accomplish tasks.

- ## The Heart Chakra

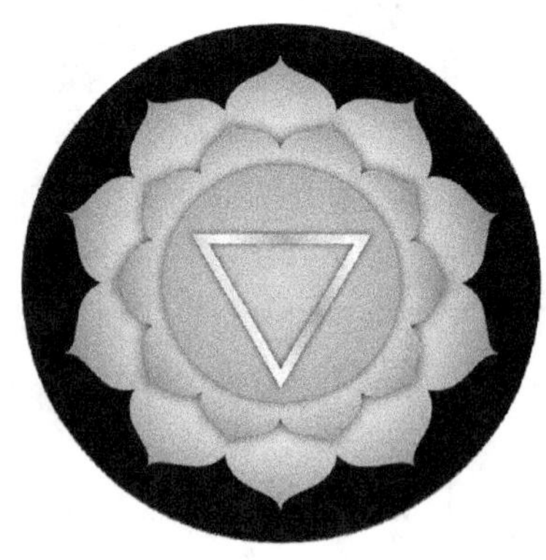

The heart chakra is related to adoration for all things that exist in this universe: generosity to strangers, sentimental love, empathy for other people, fellowship, and familial love. On the off chance that you are encountering any of the accompanying side effects, you may have an irregularity in the heart chakra: pain in your upper back or chest, tight shoulders or, on the other hand, excessively adaptable shoulders, inability to receive love or to reciprocate love, and lack of self-empathy.

- **The Throat Chakra**

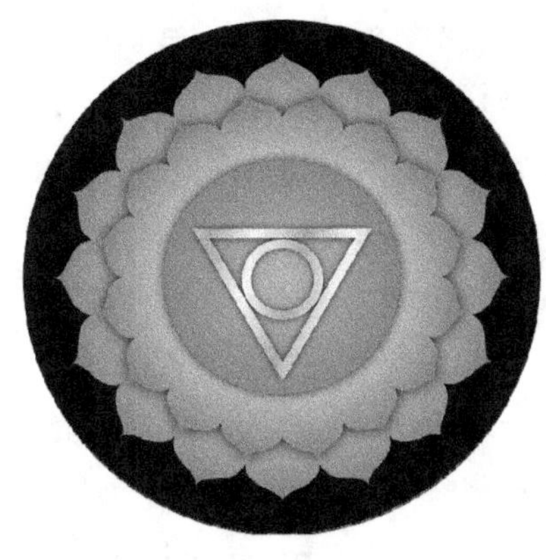

This throat chakra, which is physically situated at the throat, neck, mouth, jaw, and ears, is associated with the element sound. The throat chakra is related to the act of talking, articulation, utilizing your voice, and realizing when to remain calm or stay quiet. This chakra is identified with your capacity to talk from your heart and brain with clearness and to tune in with empathy. On the off chance that you are encountering any of the accompanying side effects, you may have an irregularity in the throat chakra: sore throat or laryngitis, jaw aches or propensity for granulating your teeth, pain or stiffness in your neck, a propensity for talking constantly and not realizing when to remain calm and stay silent, and inability to voice out their opinions.

- **The Third Eye Chakra**

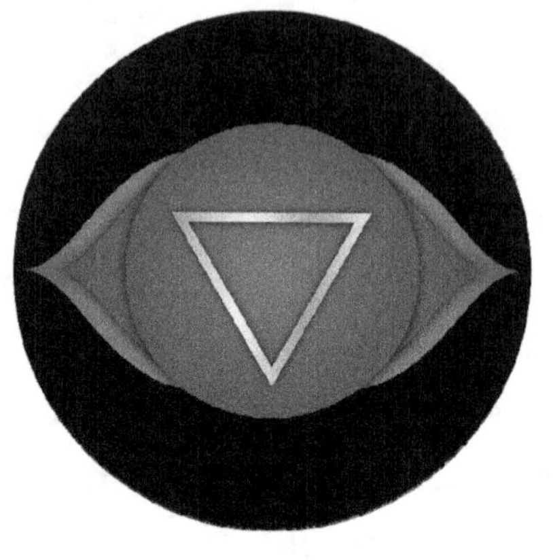

The third eye chakra is related to your instinct, creative mind, and knowledge. This chakra is likewise identified with your capacity to see profoundly inside your heart and identify the most genuine feelings. At the point when the third eye chakra is open, you see the master plan and have a positive perspective on what's to come. In the event that you are encountering any of the accompanying manifestations, you may have an irregularity in the third eye chakra: headaches, lack of direction in life, lack of motivation, hyperactiveness, and the need to overpower or dominate others just so that you can accomplish your goals.

- **The Crown Chakra**

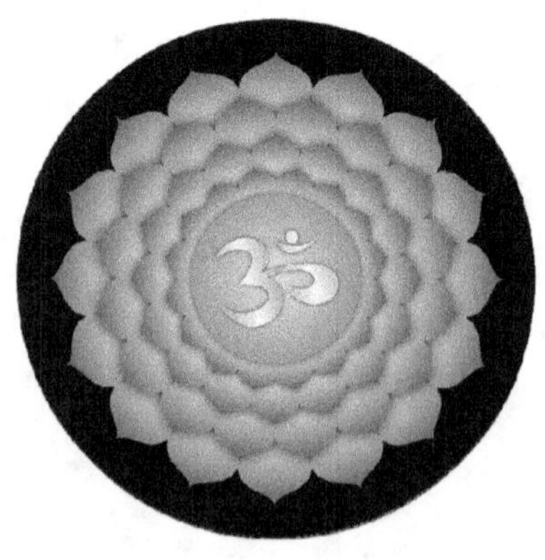

The crown chakra is related to your feelings of illumination and recognition. In the event that you are encountering any of the accompanying manifestations, you may have an irregularity in the crown chakra: headaches, inability to focus or concentrate on the job at hand, seemingly consistent dramatization in your life, inability to see past your very own little corner of the world, and inability to take on other's points of view or perspective.

The chakra framework is one approach to comprehend the human body. Indeed, even minor aggravations in the inconspicuous body can show as torment, distress, or general disharmony in your body, brain, heart, and soul. As you advance on your adventure toward equalization, euphoria, and bliss, consider checking in with your chakras routinely. Researching the chakras can be a decent way to check your entire system. Ensure that your adventure is all-natural and guided by your inner voice. If you feel like you cannot tap into that inner voice, then you're a long way to go.

Healing Remedies And Treatments For Unbalanced Chakras

Despite the fact that there are 114 chakra centers in the body, there are about seven main ones that are commonly targeted with regards to the recuperation of one's holistic health. As you know, these are the root chakra (first chakra), sacral chakra (second chakra), solar plexus chakra (third chakra), heart chakra (fourth chakra), throat chakra (fifth chakra), third eye chakra (sixth chakra), and the crown chakra (seventh chakra). The objective behind every single profound practice is to arrive at a position of harmony between soul, body, earth, and wellbeing. The following are a couple of procedures used to open and heal these chakra points.

- **Chakra Healing Through Affirmations**

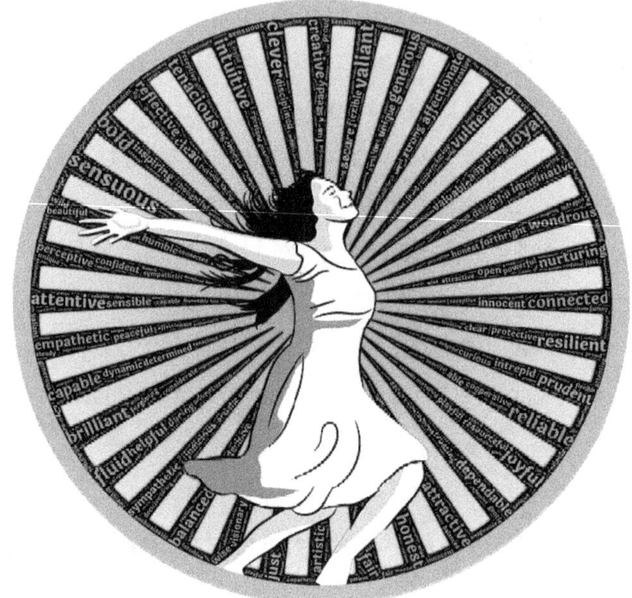

One of the amazing tools utilized for chakra healing is attestations or affirmations. These are phrases that have the capacity of fortifying and recuperating ourselves. When working with affirmations, we can concentrate on different perspectives, each one in turn. Here are a few examples for each of the different chakras:

- o The Root Chakra - "I am loaded up with modesty." and "I am sufficient as I am."

- o The Sacral Chakra - "I am brilliant and excellent in my own way." and "I am living a good life."

- o The Solar Plexus Chakra - "I acknowledge myself totally." and "I acknowledge that I have qualities and I acknowledge that I also have shortcomings."

- o The Heart Chakra - "Love is the response to everything throughout everyday life, and I give and get love unequivocally."

- o The Throat Chakra - "My considerations are accurate as to what I want to portray." and "I, in every case, convey what needs to be conveyed honestly."

- o The Third Eye Chakra - "I am wise." and "I comprehend the genuine significance of life's circumstances."

- o The Crown Chakra - "I am one with what the universe wants for me."

- **Chakra Healing Through Colors**

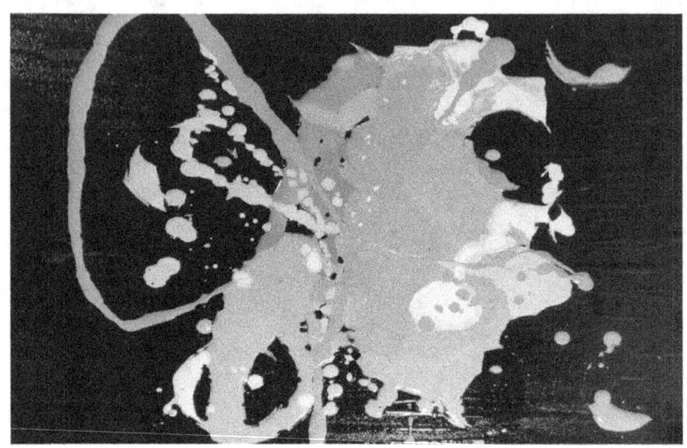

At the point when presented to various kinds of hues that all have their own set of vibrations, our physical state, feelings, and temperaments can be changed. This is because our chakra framework - the one responsible for all of these - is affected by various colors. We can rebalance the chakras by presenting our body to various hues in our homes, our nourishment, and the garments that we wear. Different approaches to ingest hues is to wear shading glasses that ingest the vibrations required in our bodies.

- **Chakra Healing Through Music**

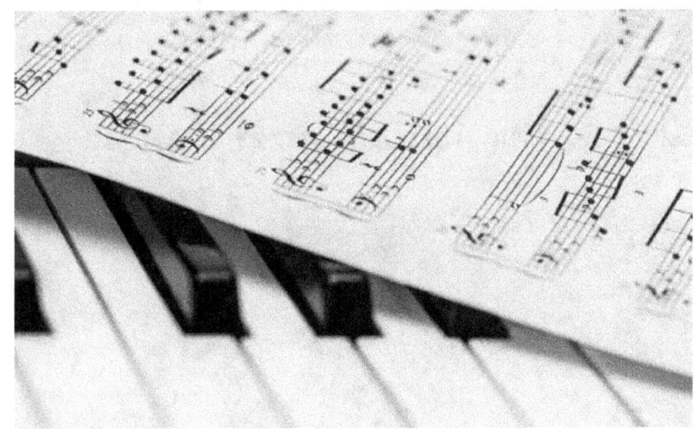

There is also such a thing called chakra balancing music. Here, healers would often use sound to balance out the seven main energy centers in our body. As explained in the previous point, each of the chakra points responds to a particular color - and you'll also learn that it responds to certain types of gemstones. Well, our chakras also respond to certain sound healing frequencies. These tunes are called the Solfeggio frequencies. Moreover, these are made up using a very old six-tone scale that is often used in ancient societies as sacred chanting and music.

When it comes to the Solfeggio frequencies, all you need to remember is that each chakra point corresponds to a musical notation - B, A, G, F, E, D, and C. The root chakra is energized by the musical notation, C. The second chakra by the musical notation, D. The solar plexus chakra is energized by the musical notation, E.

F energizes the heart chakra; the throat chakra by G; the third eye chakra by A. Finally, the crown chakra is energized by the musical notation, B.

- **Chakra Healing Through Energy Healers**

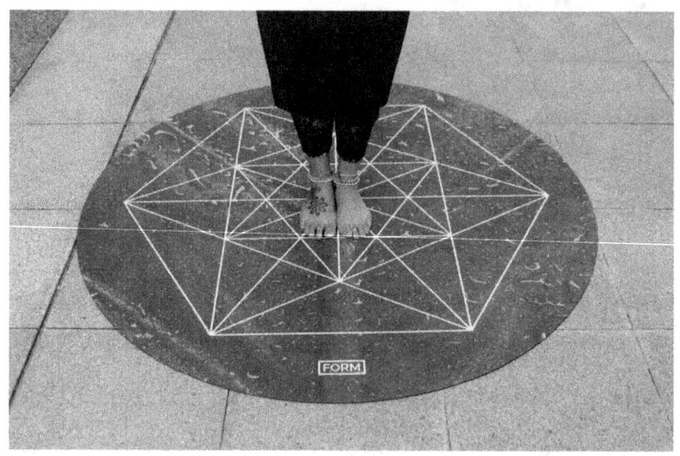

Proficient and experienced chakra healers offer administrations that analyze an individual's vitality levels in their chakra framework. In addition, they are also capable of finding and pinpointing the reasons why there is a blockage. After an exhaustive assessment, they can offer appropriate healing medications with respect to which chakra point you would like to balance or open.

- **Chakra Healing Through Stones**

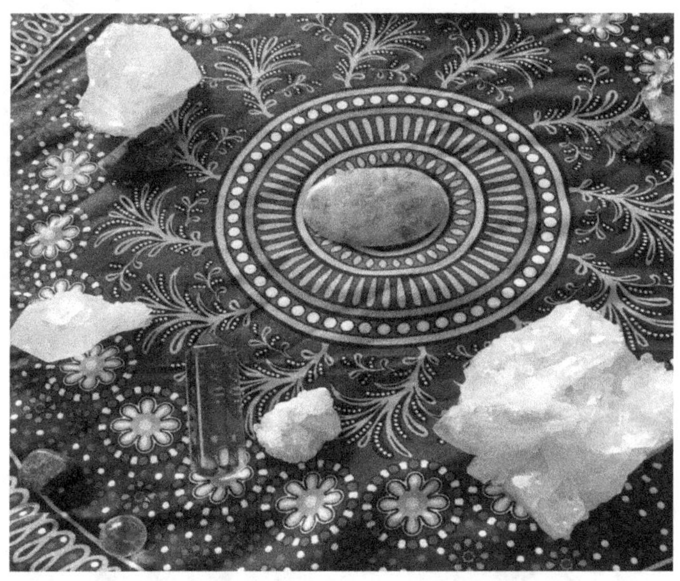

The chakra stones are known as healing precious stones that contain explicit hues and vibrations. Time and time again, we have explained how each chakra has a predefined color correspondence, and this equivalent shading can be utilized in chakra healing. Nonetheless, despite the fact that most of the stones with a specific shading will be utilized to recuperate a particular chakra, there are also a couple of stones that can be used to heal two or more chakras at once.

- **Chakra Healing Through Yoga**

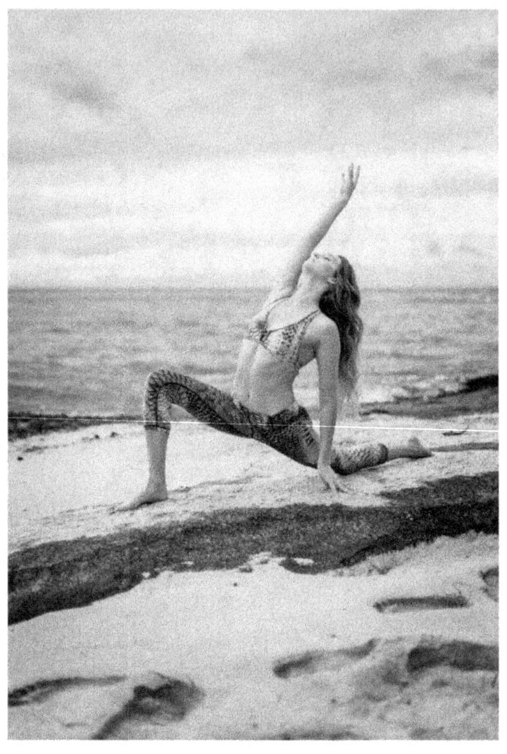

At the point when a particular wheel-of-vitality or chakra is unbalanced or blocked, it tends to prevent the Chi or Prana from discharging; thus, any development within the self is achieved. Yoga stances, on the other hand, have been deemed as a great way to counter this happenstance. Yoga has been perceived as an excellent and effective method to unblock certain chakra points to allow the flow of Chi or Prana out of the body, and for the crown chakra to start receiving the blessings from the universe.

- **Chakra Healing Through Fundamental Oils**

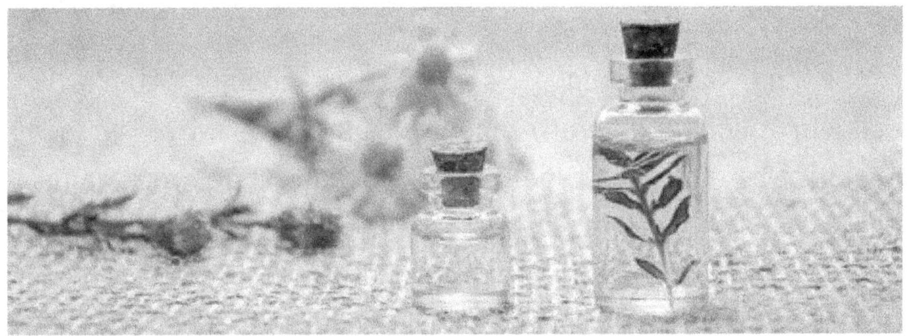

Fundamental oils additionally structure a significant piece of chakra healing and are for the most part utilized alongside chakra balancing massages. The following is a rundown of prescribed oils for each chakra:

- o First Chakra: St. Johnís Wort, Angelica, Patchouli, and Frankincense

- o Second Chakra: Orange, Neroli, Clove, Juniper, and Rosemary

- o Third Chakra: Lemon, Rosemary, Peppermint, Yarrow, and Marjoram

- o Fourth Chakra: Melissa, Rosewood, Basil, and Rose

- o Fifth Chakra: Lemongrass, Sage, and Blue chamomile

- o Sixth Chakra: Clary sage, Elemi, Spruce, and Lavender

o Seventh Chakra: Geranium, Myrrh, Gotu Kola, and Sandalwood

In the end, we couldn't stress this enough: there is a need for each and every one of you to be able to adapt accordingly to the type of technique that you want to accomplish when it comes to achieving a well-balanced chakra framework. This book will comprise of so many details regarding stances, color correspondences, gemstones or crystal correspondences, and so much more. It will definitely be overwhelming and, at some parts of the book, you will feel like it's very repetitive; this is normal because if there is one thing you should learn from chakra meditative practice is that everything is interconnected.

Notice how each of the chakra points is associated with a particular color or organ in the body. Moreover, notice how one is supposed to start from the very bottom that is the root chakra and only moving upwards toward the crown chakra, and not the other way around. Also, notice the need for each chakra color to be incorporated in what you wear, what you eat, and whatnot. Well, all of these aren't merely random rules that someone had thought up years ago. From Ancient China to some of the Southeast Asian countries to Western civilization, these methods all serve a purpose. Thus, if one of these is not functioning well - for example, if one chakra point is blocked - there is no way an individual can achieve holistic health. This is what we want you to understand when it comes to meditative practice - you need all cogs for the machine to work properly. With enough patience, all of these would soon make sense to you as the universe will definitely enlighten you with the answers that you are looking for.

Chapter 5:
Advanced Self-Healing Techniques: Healing Multiple Chakras And Awakening Your Higher Self

Step-By-Step Guided Meditation

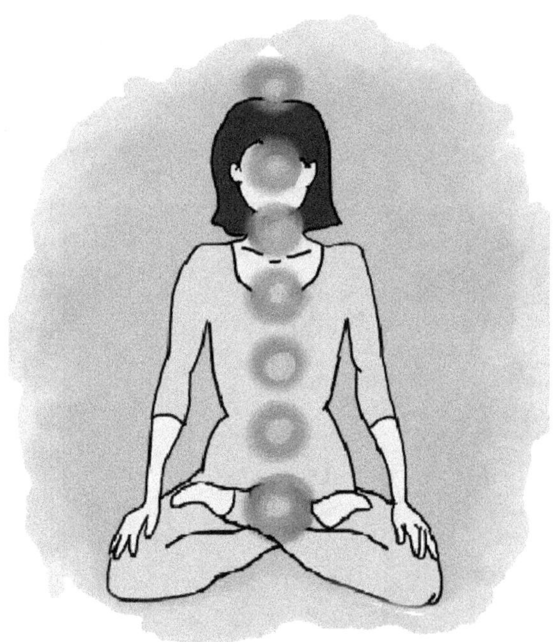

Chakra meditation includes unblocking and adjusting the progression of vitality all through your body with profound focus. By following these basic advances, you can begin the act of chakra meditation, and find its advantages over some undefined time frame. We have brushed on this topic earlier, but only to explain the correlations of colors, music, and such to the different chakras in the body. Here, we will proceed with the end goal in mind - the opening of your crown chakra and allowing the inspiration of the entire universe to enter your body, resulting in your holistic health.

1st Step - Sit in the lotus posture in a quiet spot. Inhale deeply while you loosen up your body and close your eyes.

2nd Step - Concentrate first on your root chakra, which can be located at the bottom or foundation of your spine. Envision the region shining red and being loaded up with a warm and ameliorating light.

3rd Step - Envision the light ascending to the sacral chakra. Envision the shading changing to orange, making you feel progressively sexy and alluring.

4th Step - Draw the light further up into your solar plexus chakra. Envision it changing to the color yellow; a representation for power and vitality.

5th Step - Give the light a chance to stream up to your heart and turn green, filling you with sentiments of affection and harmony.

6th Step - Further draw the light to your throat chakra. Imagine it turning into a wad of blue streams of energy. Feel the intensity of conveying everything that needs to be conveyed plainly.

7th Step - Give the light a chance to move up to your third eye chakra, which is located at your temple, and envision the shading becoming purple, filling you with instinct and expanding your mystic capacities.

8th Step - At long last, envision the light turning white as it streams up to your crown chakra. Feel your own vitality interfacing with different flows known to man.

9th Step - Inhale deeply a few times. Then, when you are ready, open your eyes and stretch.

There are those who take as long as a few minutes before they advance on to the next chakra center. For others, it would take them about half an hour before they proceed to open the other five chakras. Of course, with meditation, all of these are up to you. Do so when you are ready. You'll know when you are ready when you believe that you have managed to manifest the objectives of each chakra. For example: with the root chakra, you'll be able to advance to the second one if you feel grounded with everything that is happening in your life. If you feel that you are unsure or if you fear the future and what's to come, then it is a clear sign that you have not achieved enlightenment for the first chakra. Again, repetition and practice are key. You may want to include this is as routine to your everyday set of tasks. It's best done in the morning before you start your day. Nevertheless, you can meditate on one chakra a day or on all chakras a day - as long as you follow the steps and start with the lowest chakra up to the crown chakra.

Top Meditation Methods To Connect To The Spirit

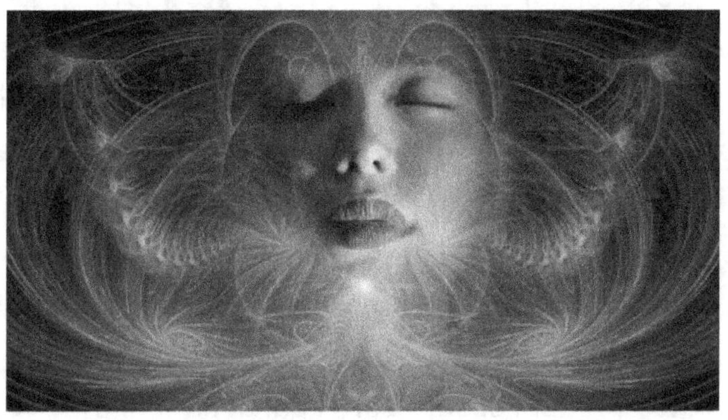

We as a whole have our very own spirit guides or guardian angels. We have guides much like that of our ancestors. There are those that have names, there are those that don't have names. It may even be possible that you've had encounters with these entities before. There are times when you are aware that whom you are interacting with are the spirit guides, yet there are times when you are completely oblivious as to their presence. In the event that you have had encounters with these entities, the stages we share below will assist you with having a much profound way of connecting with them. You'll develop your association with your spirit guides and figure out how to approach them properly should there be a need to. In the event that you haven't had encounters like these, we welcome you to keep an open mind. On the off chance that you are happy to associate with your spirit guide, these straightforward methods will help you.

This may sound a little out of the ordinary to you, and we completely understand why. Yet, we would like to assure you that all spirit guides are adoring and insightful. They exist for a reason as they are here to help you. Connecting or communicating with them will most likely be a blissful experience. These spirit guides are just here to guide you to achieve a good life or even a well-balanced chakra system. There are a lot of elements in this topic; however, the spirit guides that we approach, our guardian angels, are here to bring you only good things in life; it's just a matter of approaching them the correct way.

When you start warming up to the possibility of the existence of these spirit guides, we would like to advise you that there are various ways you may encounter their presence - even without you fully knowing it. You can encounter them as an inward inkling or a voice inside. You may hear the voice of your spirit guides or you may even observe them. In fact, there have been instances when people would claim that they saw sparkles of light either from themselves or from another person. Some would share how they may not see their spirit guides, but they can truly feel their presence. Now, the actual feeling of what their presence is like may vary from person to person. Nevertheless, if there is one thing common among their stories is that it would always be a good and positive emotion.

Now, at this point, you may already be asking the question: How do we get in contact with these spirit guides? Well, there are a number of methods to do so. But first, we would like to state its relationship with chakra meditation. You see, it's pretty simple. Your spirit guides are messengers that have been sent out by the universe to guide you in your journey. At least, that's the way we see it. If you are feeling lost or if you are unable to unblock a particular chakra point, you may want to call upon your spirit guide to help you with a certain roadblock. Nevertheless, even if you do not call upon them knowingly, they may grant you their presence at times of need. Of course, it's more advisable to be able to call unto them when you truly need them so that you are better able to develop a healthier relationship and a better chance of achieving holistic health.

With all of these in mind, let's begin with the most basic step - something that you may already be familiar with - finding a place of solitude. As you may notice as you progress with your reading that most of the items here would be similar to the step-by-step meditative practice you have learned earlier. A nice and quiet place is a great place to give your mind some time away from the hustle and bustle of your daily routine. You can even play some gentle music or light some scented candles. We would like to remind you that you need to achieve a relaxed state, but not too relaxed that you'll fall asleep. Use the type of candle or music that makes you feel invigorated as it will prevent you from falling asleep. The next step would comprise of selecting the proper position - lying down, standing up, or sitting down are some of the common stances people prefer when trying to contact their spirit guides. Moreover, before you begin, it is important to turn off all devices that may disturb you from your reverie, which means turn off your cellphones or put it into silent mode if you're using it for music. Similar to your meditative practice, be sure that you are focusing on your breathing. It will help you keep your mind calm and relaxed.

Now, the next step is a variation from what you would normally do when you're trying to transfer the energy from one chakra point to the other. Instead of envisioning a white light or a light that is associated with a particular chakra, envision a gold shimmering aura surrounding your very existence. Moreover, instead of imagining the vitality coming from within you, imagine the exact opposite and try to visualize the gold aura slowly enveloping you with its power. It is important that you have your set of questions or requests ready at hand. We don't mean that you write them down on a piece of paper, but if it helps, you can do that as well. Do remember that if you are asking a question, the answer may come immediately or in a few days or weeks - or longer. Now, you may or may not feel something as you focus on the gold aura and your breathing. The important thing is that you were able to manifest the questions out into the universe. It has left your subconscious mind, passed through your conscious mind, and traveled out into the universe. All you need to do now is to simply wait for the answer. The answer that you are looking for will, of course, come from the universe. By this time, you should have already achieved a well-established chakra system because, as you know, the universe will pass the message - in this case, answers - to you via your crown chakra.

If you're having a hard time thinking of the questions to ask, make a rundown of the five to ten greatest things you need assistance with. You can do this now, or you can return to this activity subsequent to line up with your time for reflection. Tune in to that inner voice and let the considerations come through. This is the universe's way of communicating with you. When you have made this rundown, offer up all that you need assistance with and welcome in the spirit guide with the most elevated truth and empathy to uncover arrangements. Moreover, don't forget to thank them once you are done. At this point, you can sit in reflection for five, ten, or 20 minutes. This can be an extremely basic contemplation. You can just focus on your breathing, getting to be aware of the sounds and sensations around you or, you can rehash a mantra quietly, which is one of the most preferred approaches by people.

For most individuals who have never attempted any kind of meditative practice before, it might be hard to get a grip on exactly what the advantages are in relation to this activity. Meditation has been around for a large number of years and has been esteemed for this long because it works - it can really change your body, your brain, your spirit, and your whole life on the off chance that you are ready to make yourself available to it. In any case, one of the principal reasons that individuals neglect to begin with profound contemplation is just that they don't have the foggiest idea of how to begin doing it. On the off chance that you are keen on encountering a portion of the extraordinary advantages of contemplation and meditation; however, you aren't sure where to start, then these tips can help and enable you to comprehend not just the advantages that you will begin experiencing with basic meditative practice, yet see how to truly incorporate this practice into your daily routine so you can start to perceive how it can transform you as a whole.

Before you begin with your meditative journey, it is critical to comprehend what the advantages of this practice are or, to put it plainly, why you are doing this every single day. If you are not convinced that there is a purpose to this practice, then you might as well stop now because it won't take you anywhere. The more you comprehend the "why" of meditative practice, the simpler it will be to remain engaged and committed to the artistic expression and to truly work at making it a part of your daily routine. Contemplating ought to be a piece of your day by day custom, much like brushing your teeth. You brush your teeth every day, or even at various times each day, on the grounds that simply brushing your teeth once wouldn't generally do anything for you. A similar mentality ought to be applied to meditative practice. You have to do it routinely so as to experience its benefits. Meditative practice should be tied in with being aware of where you are on the planet and getting to be available at the present time. This means that you are not caught up with a memory that had happened to your five years ago nor with what is to happen five years from now. You have to be absolutely mindful of where you are and of your surroundings to be really present at the moment. This can take some time but it's definitely possible.

Breathing is one of the most significant aspects of meditative practice, and it is crucial that you figure out how to concentrate on your breathing so that you can move forward with your meditative journey. Try to take in long and full breaths every time you reflect. It also helps if you can envision the air coursing through your body, in and out through your lungs, and through your nose. The more centered you can remain around your breathing, the better. Envision your breaths as being profound, purifying, and therapeutic breaths that can help you take in the greatness around you and exhale the negativity in your life. Remember, visualization is key. We've talked about it in the earlier chapters of this book because it is one of the basic principles when attempting to achieve mindfulness. As you keep on becoming acclimated to your breath, you can take a chance at focusing on a mantra or even a positive idea, word, or attestation. You can likewise have a go at murmuring "Om" as you breathe in and out. From that point, you simply need to rehash this procedure as much as you can. It is important to start small, especially if you are new to all of these. In the event that you can't remain still and be centered for the entire ten minutes, then simply start meditating for only five minutes and move your way up to longer periods of meditative practice. Again, the more you practice, the simpler it will be.

Various Meditation Poses You Can Use

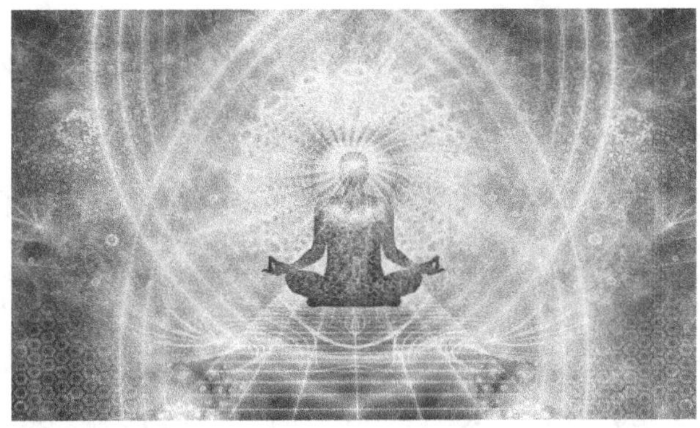

Meditative practice doesn't have a one-size-fits-all step-by-step process to follow. There are many varieties and strategies that are accessible to you. Yet, you don't have to peruse each book to determine what works best for you. You simply need to try various stances, postures, and strategies until you find the right one that works for you. You'll know that it's the right one when you are able to concentrate on your visualization practice. Another thing most people fail to realize when it comes to meditative practice is that it can be done whenever and wherever. Regardless of whether you're a beginner or a well-advanced student, it's imperative to remain adaptable in your methodology. Making a routine that works for you is critical, and you'll likely alter and change your training to suit your developing needs; this is absolutely normal. With that in mind, we would like to present to you some of the more common meditation poses. You can start your journey to finding the right meditative stance here:

- **Sitting Meditation Poses**

You can undoubtedly ruminate while sitting in a seat or on the ground, making this ideal for early afternoon meditative practice. The best part is that if you have a place of solitude at work, you can easily sneak in a 10-minute meditation. You can ruminate at work or while you're traveling. Moreover, if you want to truly accomplish a successful meditation session, you need to get in the correct position; sit in your seat or the ground with a straight back and with your feet level on the floor - if you're using a chair. They should frame a 90-degree angle with your knees. You may need to also slightly sit at the edge of the seat so that you're not slouching. Sit upright so your head and neck are in accordance with your spine. You may put a pad behind your lower back or under your hips for added help. In the event that you aren't sure how to manage your hands, you can lay them on your knees or put them in your lap.

o The Quarter Lotus Sitting Position

To achieve this, you need to sit with your legs loosely crossed over one another. Both of your feet should be resting just below the opposite knee or thigh. This is often called as the Indian Seat. Most beginners would start with this meditative pose.

o   The Half Lotus Sitting Position

This is a variation from the above-mentioned. One of your legs is crossed with one foot laying on the opposite thigh. The other foot is then extended forward.

o   The Full Lotus Sitting Position

Now, the full lotus sitting position may sometimes be mistaken for the quarter lotus sitting position, but to distinguished the two, keep in mind that the full lotus sitting position requires that both of your legs are resting on the opposite thigh.

o   The Burmese Sitting Position

In the event that you can't sit with your legs crossed, that is fine. Simply sit with the two feet laying on the floor in this casual position, otherwise known as Sukhasana or the Easy Pose.

o   The Seiza Sitting Position

Rather than sitting with your legs crossed, you can also stoop and place a pad or yoga mats between your legs. This customary reflection stance is basically a propped-up Virasana, which is known as the Hero Pose, or Vajrasana, which is known as the Thunderbolt Pose.

- **Standing Meditation Poses**

In case you're more comfortable with standing up, have a go at a standing meditation pose. To do this, stand tall with your feet apart. Your shoulder should also fall naturally to the side. Now, do note that some well-advanced students would tend to execute certain positions with their hands but, for now, it's better to start with something normal.

When you're in position, somewhat bend your knees - as if you're sitting down on an imaginary stool. Envision your vitality moving upwards to the crown of your head every time you breathe in. For added assistance, you can also place your hands on your stomach with the goal of feeling your breath traveling through your body.

- **Resting or Lying Down Meditation Poses**

You may also want to lie down when meditating as this is one of the most comfortable positions known to most beginners. However, you must not fall asleep. It is important to still be aware of what you're doing as you meditate. Nevertheless, to do this, lie on your back with your arms stretched out near your body. Your feet ought to be aligned with your hips, and your toes should be pointed outward.

On the off chance that this is awkward, adjust the posture to help you release some tension on your lower

138

back. Put a cushion underneath your knees to somewhat lift them while lying down. You can likewise bend your knees and firmly place your feet on the ground.

Do remember that your pose is basic to meditative practice, yet you can adopt various strategies to suit your needs. It's critical to begin in an agreeable spot, with the goal that you can easily move your body accordingly. You may find that keeping up a particular stance causes you to set a positive expectation or resolve for your training. When you return to the stance or position, you can help yourself to remember the real reason you're doing all of these — to be available, to feel loose, or whatever else you may require.

- **How To Do The Seven-Point Meditation Posture**

The seven-point meditation posture is a way to go about it when you are used to sitting while, at the same time, meditating. There are seven rules that you can use to accurately execute this position. Obviously, you're free to change whatever doesn't work for you. Approach the stance in a similar way that you would approach your meditation process. Your body is effectively connected with the rest of yourself, yet there is a delicate quality to it if you want to achieve holistic health.

1. Sitting

Contingent upon how adaptable your hips are, you can sit in the quarter, half, or full lotus position. You can sit "leg over leg" with your hips raised higher than your heels by sitting on a yoga mat, towel, cushion, or seat. You can utilize a pad to get support in many positions. It's imperative to pick something that is agreeable so you can concentrate on your meditative practice.

2. Spine

Regardless of how you sit, your spine ought to be as straight as could be allowed. On the off chance that you tend to sluggard forward or do something in reverse, right now is an ideal opportunity to delicately remind yourself to return into the right stance. Even though meditative postures are very relaxing and comfortable, you need to be aware and conscious of everything that you are doing. Find a stance that is comfortable, but not too comfortable that you'll fall asleep or lose focus.

Keep your focus on your spine as you breathe in and out the air that fills your lungs. Lift your body up and protract your spine with each breath. Feel the line of vitality that goes from the bottom or foundation of your spine out through the top of your head. Keeping your spine straight will assist you with staying alert.

3. Hands

The most basic rule for the hands is to lay them on your thighs with your palms facing down. Keeping your hands put down is said to be useful for establishing the chakra points and helping your body to loosen up so that the Chi or Prana can easily pass through the various points.

You can also stack your hands in your lap with your palms looking up. To do this, place your right hand over your left hand with your thumbs delicately in contact with each other. This hand position is said to produce more warmth and energy. It's perfect for when you want to wake up a chakra point. On the other hand, if you are trying to visualize the Chi or Prana transferring from one center to the other, then you will have better luck with the first-hand position.

4. Shoulders

Keep your shoulders loose and comfortable. If you feel tense, try to loosen up first before actually starting your meditative practice. This is an important step because your ultimate goal is to awaken your root chakra, then move that same energy from the bottom or foundation of your spine to the top of your head. Nevertheless, if you are too tensed, then it may add to the blockage of certain chakra points. Thus, the Chi or Prana would not be able to pass through. Also, if you think about it, this position or stance helps keep your heart open and your back firm, which may help your spine as well.

During your meditative practice, check your stance every now and then. Even if you start to drift away or your mind began to wander, try to slowly bring yourself back and resume the correct stance. Again, it is important that you should not feel forced when doing this. You must not exert too much energy. Relax and don't stress about not getting it right the first time. Remember that chakra meditation is a process. No one gets it right the first time. You'll eventually perfect it once you start to incorporate it into your routine. Think of this process as a journey. Opening the crown chakra may be the goal, but the journey is necessary so that you can understand what it truly means to achieve holistic health - and actually achieve it. With that in mind, be sure that your spine is straight and drawn to the highest points of your shoulders. It should fall down gently and away from your ears.

5. Jawline

You can fix how you situate your jawline by noticing how your neck is situated. Again, if you are feeling tense, try to relax a bit. What we are trying to achieve here is a natural position that keeps you awake and mindful of every body part. Accurately situating your jawline encourages you to keep up your stance. Keep your face loose and your neck will follow through. You may find that turning the edges of your face up marginally discharges any pressure in the face.

6. Jaw

Attempt to discharge any strain you're holding in your jaw. It might be useful to keep your jaw marginally open as you press your tongue against the top of your mouth. This consequently loosens up the jaw, takes into account clear breathing, and hinders any gulping tendencies. You can also complete a couple of overstated yawns before you ponder to extend your jaw and discharge strain.

7. Eyes

The vast majority think that it is simpler to ponder with their eyes closed. Abstain from pressing your eyes shut if you are to meditate like this - just allow your eyelids to fall naturally. Delicately shutting them will enable you to keep your face, eyes, and eyelids loose, which is an important aspect of meditative practice. There are also those who would rather meditate with open eyes. Oftentimes, they want to meditate outside so that they can observe things that are part of nature as it relaxes them, allowing them to concentrate on the Chi or Prana in the body. Moreover, some would simply focus on the floor or the lining on the ceiling.

Just remember to keep your face loose and abstain from squinting.

Finally, choose what direction you'll think before you start meditating, so you're not constantly changing your view in between open and shut eyes. This can be perplexing and it can upset the progression of your meditative practice.

Crystals For Chakra Balancing

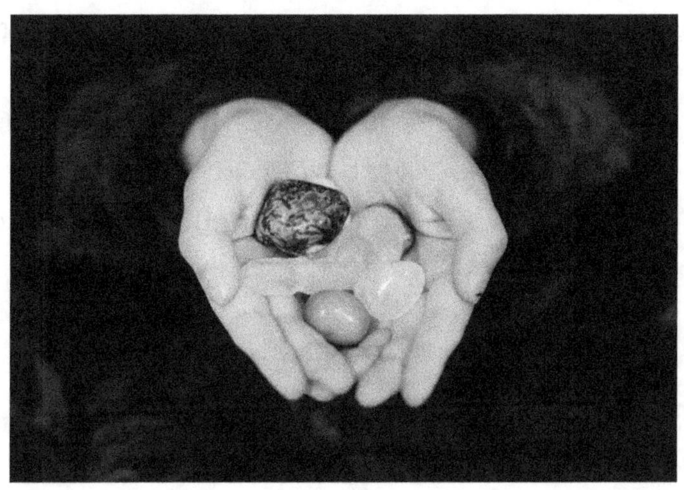

- **The Root Chakra**

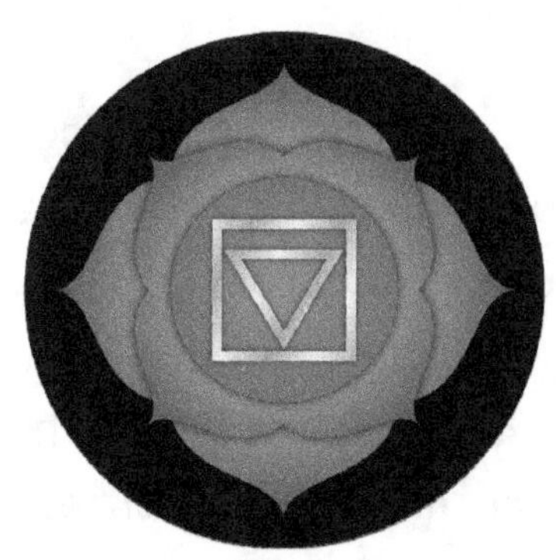

When you are meditating on your root chakra, it is best to use one or several stones. Here's a list to help you choose a particular healing crystal to guide you on achieving a balanced root chakra: Black Obsidian, Red Zincite, Smoky Quartz, Hematite, Garnet Spinel, Zircon, and Black Tourmaline. All of these represent stability, physical energy, grounding, security, and will; characteristics associated with the root chakra.

- **The Sacral Chakra**

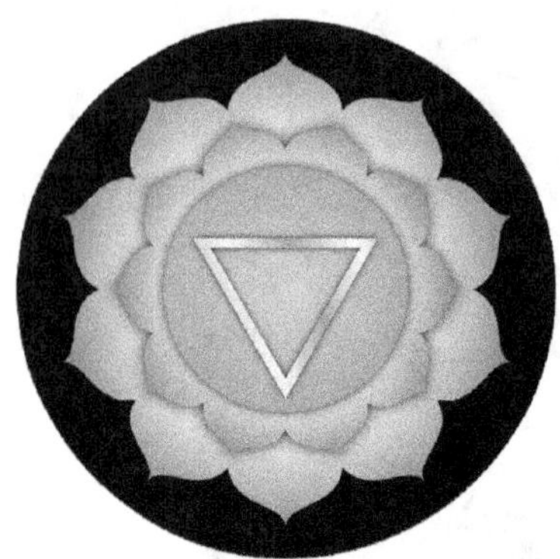

When you are meditating on your sacral chakra, it is best to use one or several stones. Here's a list to help you choose a particular healing crystal to guide you on achieving a balanced sacral chakra: Vanadinite, Carnelian, Blue-green Fluorite, Copper, Imperial Topaz, Blue-green Turquoise, and Orange Calcite. All of these represent sexuality, reproduction, emotion, desire, creativity, and intuition; characteristics associated with the sacral chakra.

- **The Solar Plexus Chakra**

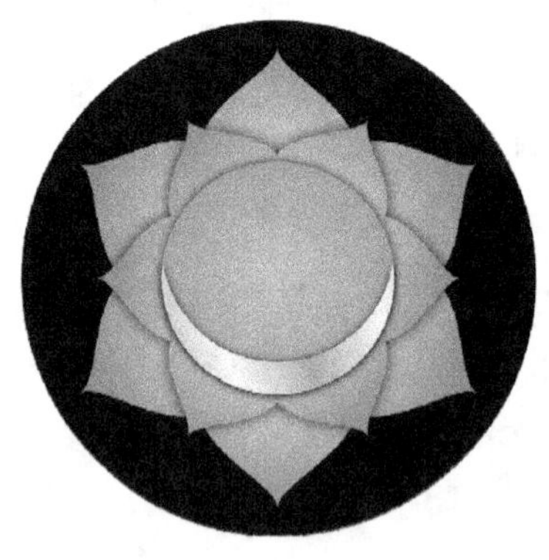

When you are meditating on your solar plexus chakra, it is best to use one or several stones. Here's a list to help you choose a particular healing crystal to guide you on achieving a balanced solar plexus chakra: Gold Tigereye, Yellow Apatite, Golden Calcite, Yellow Jasper, Amber, and Citrine. All of these represent protection or one's protectiveness, personal power, intellect, and ambition; characteristics associated with the solar plexus chakra.

146

- **The Heart Chakra**

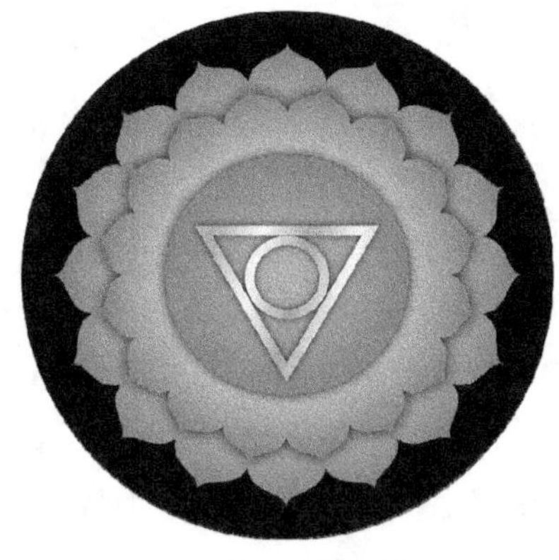

When you are meditating on your heart chakra, it is best to use one or several stones. Here's a list to help you choose a particular healing crystal to guide you on achieving a balanced heart chakra: Rose Quartz, Jade, Green Aventurine, Lepidolite, Rosasite, Pink or Rubellite Tourmaline, Cobaltian Calcite, Vesuvianite, Watermelon Tourmaline, Malachite, and Pink Danburite. All of these represent emotional balance, universal consciousness, compassion, and love; characteristics associated with the heart chakra.

- **The Throat Chakra**

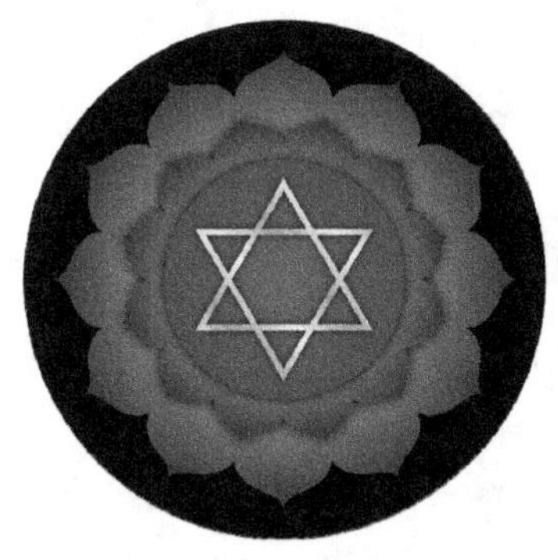

When you are meditating on your throat chakra, it is best to use one or several stones. Here's a list to help you choose a particular healing crystal to guide you on achieving a balanced throat chakra: Blue Kyanite Chrysocolla, Sodalite, Celestite, Blue Chalcedony, Angelite, Aquamarine, Blue Calcite, Blue Turquoise, and Amazonite. All of these represent diving guidance, expression, and communication center; characteristics associated with the throat chakra.

- **The Third Eye Chakra**

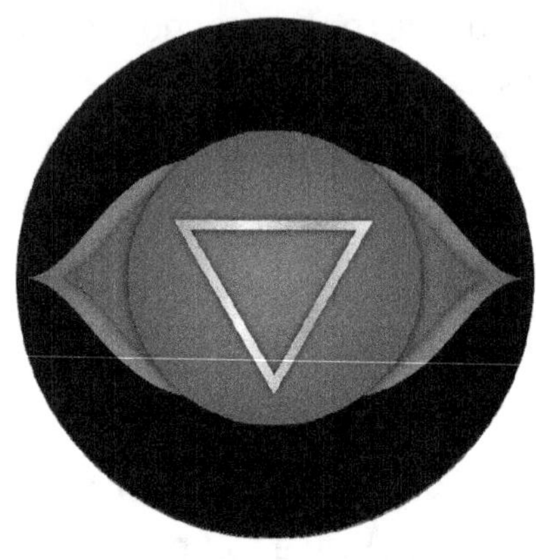

When you are meditating on your third eye chakra, it is best to use one or several stones. Here's a list to help you choose a particular healing crystal to guide you on achieving a balanced third eye chakra: Tanzanite, Lapis Lazuli, and Azurite. All of these represent spiritual awareness, intuition, psychic power, and light; characteristics associated with the third eye chakra.

- **The Crown Chakra**

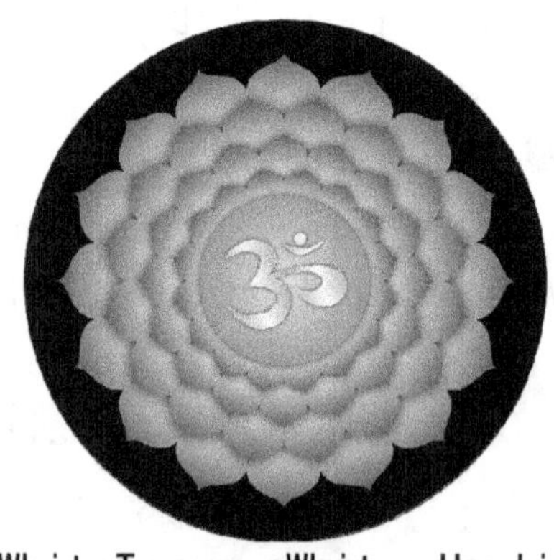

When you are meditating on your crown chakra, it is best to use one or several stones. Here's a list to help you choose a particular healing crystal to guide you on achieving a balanced crown chakra: Selenite, Amethyst, WhiteTopaz, White Howlite, Apophyllite, Herkimer Diamond, White Danburite, White Calcite, White Hemimor-

phite, and Quartz Crystal. All of these represent enlightenment, energy, perfection, and cosmic consciousness; characteristics associated with the crown chakra.

Food For Your Chakras

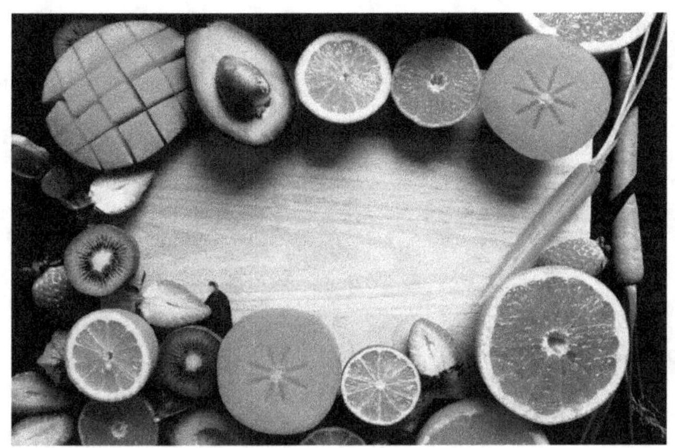

- **The Root Chakra**

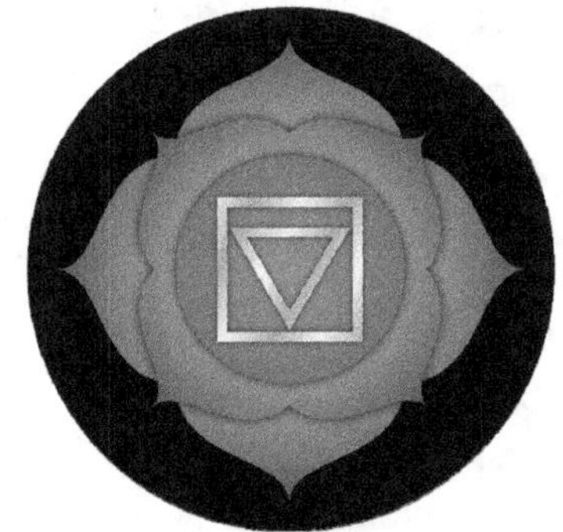

If you want to balance your root chakra, think of its correspond-ing color - red! Moreover, since this chakra is called the "root chakra," then you may have guessed that foods like garlic, onions, beets, radishes, parsnips, potatoes, and carrots should be on top of your grocery list. In addition, you can also add foods that are rich in protein like peanut butter, soy food items, tofu, beans, meats, and eggs. If you're going to eat meat, opt for lean meats. Also, the flavors that suit this chakra point are a pepper, paprika, chives, and cayenne.

- **The Sacral Chakra**

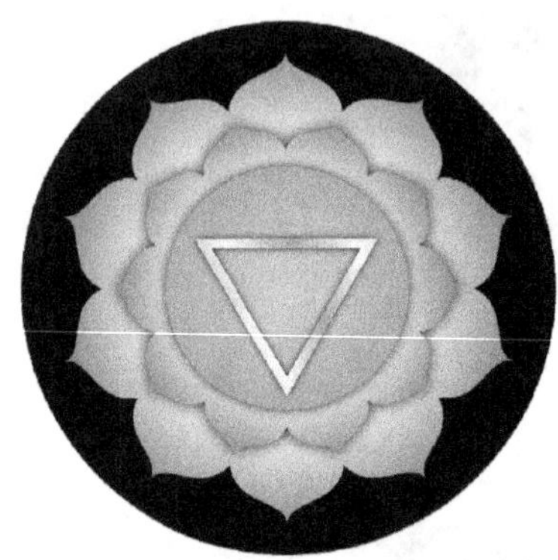

Alluding to the sacral chakra, which is situated at the navel, it is constantly associated with the color of orange. Thus, you may want to eat foods that are orange in color. This chakra is also related to everything enthusiastic and innovative. A sound sacral chakra consistently helps control and equalize one's life. Opt for more organic products like coconut, mangos, melons, and strawberries. Indeed, even nectar and nuts are suggested for helping you with sacral chakra meditation. With respect to flavors, vanilla, sesame seeds, as well as cinnamon, help to support this chakra. Also, try to add to your grocery list, carrots, apricots, peaches, foods that are rich in Omega-3s, various kinds of nuts, salmon, flax, and walnuts.

- **The Solar Plexus Chakra**

The solar plexus chakra tries to accomplish balance in confidence issues and instinctive aptitudes. Consume more grains like oats, rice, flaxseed, and sunflower seeds. If you are going to eat rice, opt for brown rice. Try to also accustom yourself to adding rye, beans, and spelt to your daily meals. Drink more milk; eat more cheese; consume more yogurt. Fennel, chamomile, cumin, mint, gin-

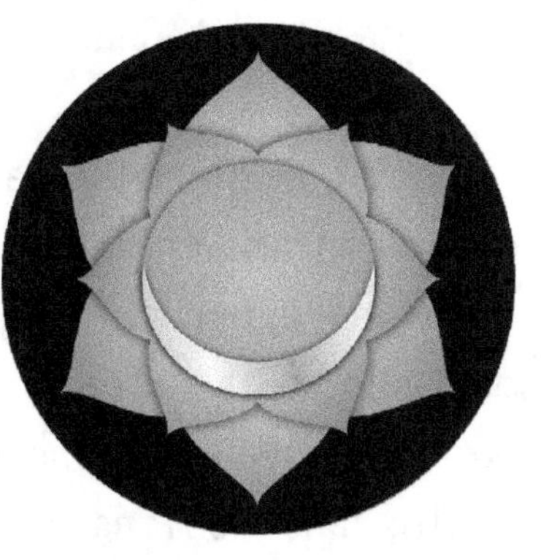

ger, and turmeric can also help with healing the solar plexus chakra, as well as foods that can provide you with sustainable energy and crucial fiber.

- **The Heart Chakra**

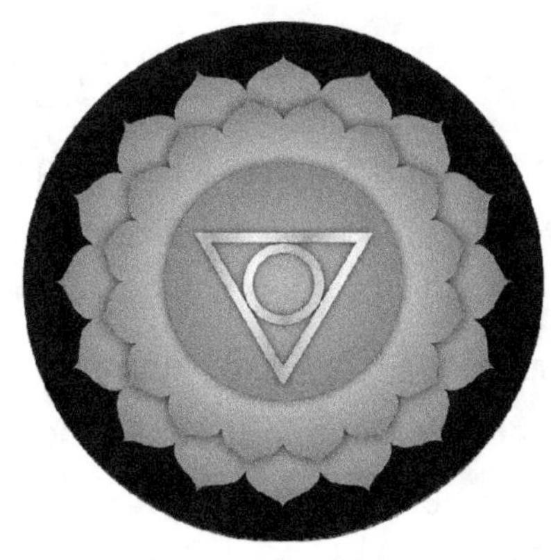

Psychological mistreatment and shock can be harmful to the seat of affection, the heart chakra. Guarantee that this chakra is consistently bal-anced by consuming green and raw foods. Think organic! Help the healing procedure by nour-ishing this chakra point with greens like broccoli, cabbage, cauliflower, celery, spinach, dandelion greens, and kale. On another note, green teas additionally maintain this particular chakra in great condition and zest it up with cilantro, basil, or thyme.

- ## The Throat Chakra

To keep the throat chakra balanced, consume fluids like water, organic product juices, and
homegrown teas. Teas are very
good as they are considered as
soothing and healing liquids, as
well as lemon water and honey.
Healing foods to be consumed are

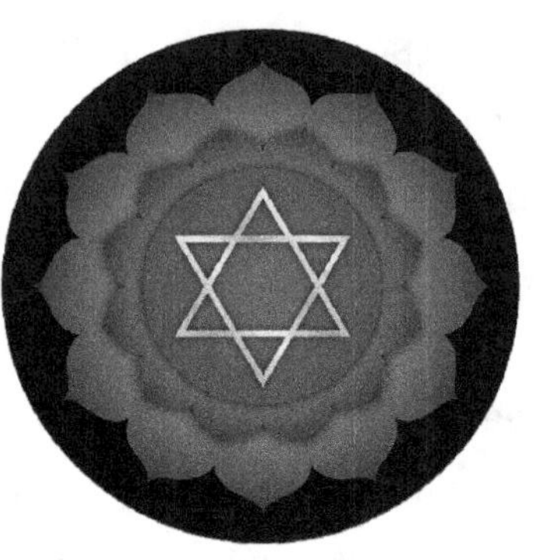

as follows: apples, plums, pears, and other foods that
are equipped with antioxidants, vitamins, and sources
of fiber.

- ## The Third Eye Chakra

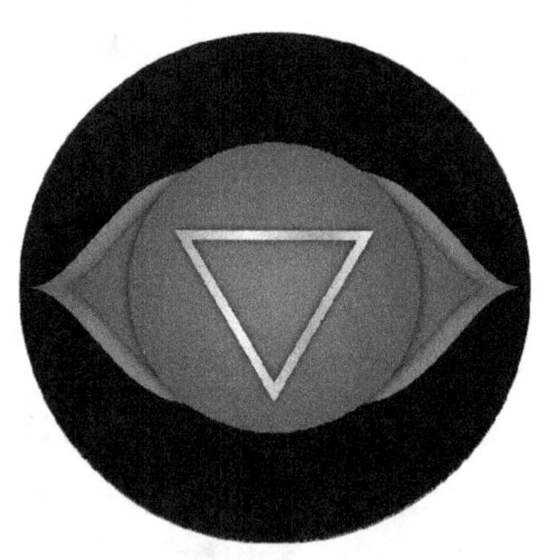

Prominently known as Ajna, the
third eye chakra is situated
in the focal point of the head
or temple. It's the seat of
intelligence and understanding. It keeps things in con-
text. Dull pale blue organic
products like blueberries,
blackberries, and raspberries
aid in keeping this particular chakra focused. Even
grape juice or wine, alongside flavors such as poppy
seeds, are viewed as ideal for this particular chakra.

- **The Crown Chakra**

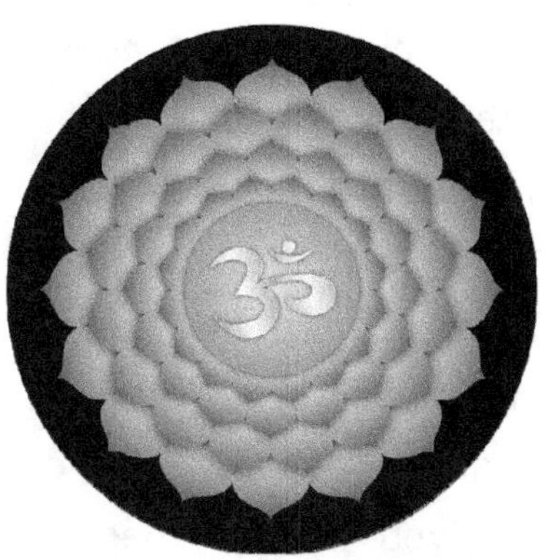

This is an important chakra point as it opens up other-worldly correspondences with the universe. It's regularly drawn or portrayed as a lotus blossoming and opening itself up to the world. Incense and smirching herbs like juniper, frankincense, copal, myrrh, and sage are best used when you are meditating on this energy center. Also, detoxifying and fasting are activities said to be useful for the advancement of this chakra.

In the end, we would like to ensure that everything presented in this book should serve as your guide, but must not all must be strictly implemented. We couldn't stress this enough - when it comes to chakra meditation, you must allow yourself to feel comfortable with yourself and with what is happening around you. This is the only way you can be honest and truthful as to how you really feel. If you are more honest about the things in your life, you'll be able to see things clearly. A good example as to what we're talking about is your stance when meditation. Of course, the most basic stance is sitting down, but there are those who prefer standing up or lying down. Moreover, there are also certain rules mentioned in this book that needs to be followed, such as the need to start at the bottom -

with the root chakra - going up to the crown chakra. Lastly, we would like to provide you with a final note that achieving mindful and holistic health will take time. However, it doesn' t mean that you should easily give up if, for the first time you' ve experienced meditative practice, did not notice any change in you. Remember that the benefits of chakra meditation will be brought to you by the universe gradually. Consistently be aware of your surroundings and it may come up to you when you least expect it.

Conclusion

Thank for making it through to the end of *"Chakra Healing For Beginners: A Complete Guide To Balance The Power Of Chakra Through Self-Healing Techniques In Order To Attract Positive Energy And Discover The Benefits Of Your Third Eye Awakening."*, let's hope that you were able to remember some of the key points in this book, starting with the fact that meditative practice takes time. It will allow you to truly be in the moment and not worry about both the past and the future, but focus on the present. Moreover, self-healing and the act of achieving holistic health is a process itself that will take time. Thus, you will need patience so that you are better able to distinguish any progress and truly see how far you have come since the start of your meditative journey. Hopefully, this book was able to provide you with insights as to the basic aspects of chakra meditation, the many misconceptions about this ancient practice, the expectations people often get when they hear chakra, chakra framework, or chakra meditation, and such. Truly, we have created and published this with the intention of spreading the knowledge on chakras. Once you have completely opened yourself up to the possibility of holistic health through chakra meditation, it will change you - not immediately, but gradually, and that's how it's supposed to be.

Of course, your chakra meditative journey does not end here. We have also created two other books focusing on chakra meditative practice but on a more specific area. You'll find that as soon as you start to get the hang of all of the practices we have mentioned in this book, you'll start to seek more challenges and poses. You'll even start to notice a change in your approach towards particular techniques - and that's a good thing because change is inevitable. You need to be constantly evolving and challenging yourself until you have successfully opened up your crown chakra. To achieve this level of enlightenment, you would need more than just the basics of chakra meditation.

Nevertheless, we would like to request from you a review on Amazon regarding your experience with this book.